total health
for children

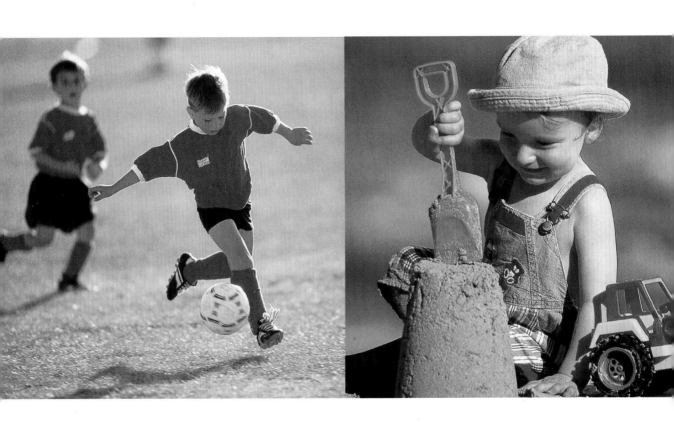

total
health
for children

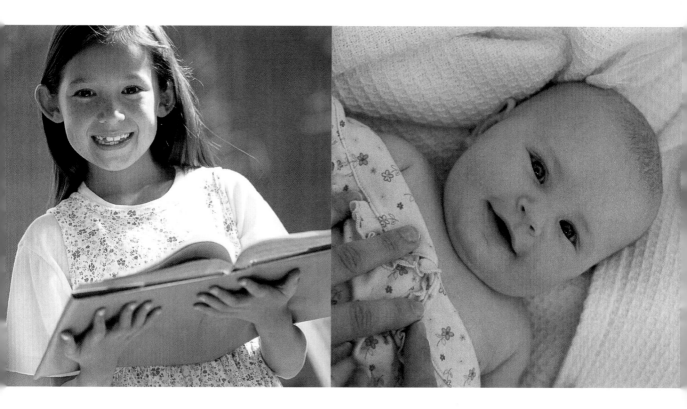

Every parent's guide to keeping your child well
and knowing what to do when illness strikes

June Thompson Sue Hubberstey Jan Hurst
Nigel Perryman Jenny Sutcliffe Nicola McClure Patsy Westcott
CONSULTANT EDITORS David Elliman Helen Bedford

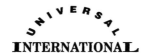

UNIVERSAL
INTERNATIONAL

A Marshall Edition
Conceived, edited and designed by Marshall Editions Ltd
The Orangery, 161 New Bond Street, London W1Y 9PA

First published in Australia and New Zealand in 2000 by
UNIVERSAL INTERNATIONAL
The Phoenix, 4th Floor, 7-9 Merriwa Street, Gordon, NSW 2072, Australia
Fax: 61 (02) 9418 4997   Email: Uni_Int@tpg.com.au

CIP information for this book is available from the National Library of Australia
Originated in PICA Colour Separation Pte. Printed and bound in Portugal by Printer Portuguesa
ISBN 1-876142-94-4

Project Editor Theresa Lane
Project Art Editor Siân Williams
Editor Gwen Rigby
Design Assistants Keith Banbury, Imran Ghoorbin, Lee Riches
Editorial Assistant Dan Green
Copy Editor Lindsay McTeague
Indexer Caroline S. Sheard
Managing Editor Anne Yelland
Managing Art Editors Patrick Carpenter, Helen Spencer
Editorial Director Ellen Dupont
Art Director Dave Goodman
Picture Editor Su Alexander
DTP Editor Lesley Gilbert
Editorial Coordinator Ros Highstead
Production Nikki Ingram

10 9 8 7 6 5 4 3 2

Picture credits: *l*=left; *r*=right; *t*=top; *b*=bottom; *c*=centre. **Front cover:**
t ZEFA-Stockmarket, *bl* Corbis/Bruce Burkhardt, *bc* The Stock Market,
br Joe Bator/Stock Market. **Back cover:** *t* Laura Wickenden, *bl* Julian Calder/ Tony
Stone Images, *bc* The Stock Market, *br* CNRI/Science Photo Library.

Note: Every effort has been taken to ensure that all information in this book is correct
and compatible with national standards generally accepted at the time of publication.
This book is not intended to replace consultation with your doctor or other healthcare
professional or to replace professional first aid training. The authors and publisher
disclaim any liability for loss, injury or damage incurred as a consequence, directly or
indirectly, of the use and application of the contents of this book.

Note: The terms "he" and "she", used in alternate articles,
refer to people of both sexes, unless a topic or sequence
of photographs applies only to a male or female.

Foreword

Raising a child is one of the most rewarding of life's experiences, but it can have its trials and tribulations. All parents want what is best for their child, but it can be difficult to know how to care for her and keep her healthy. When does a temperature warrant a telephone call to the doctor? What is the best way to wash your toddler's hair? What should you do if your child is being bullied at school?

Total Health for Children covers every aspect of a child's health and development – from newborn to 12 years of age. There is expert advice on basic childcare, from bathing a baby to weaning her; what to do if she is sick, as well as how to prevent her from getting ill; how to cope with a child's emotions, including temper tantrums and stress; how to help a child with special needs, whether she has a hearing problem or a learning difficulty; and what to do in an emergency, from treating a burn to helping a child who is choking. There is also advice to guide you on a child's progress, along with information on how the body systems work, which will help you understand why things can sometimes go wrong.

David Ellinan

Helen Bedford.

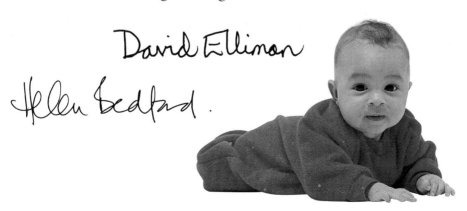

Contents

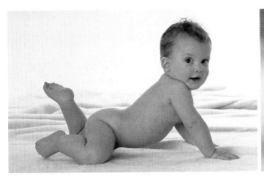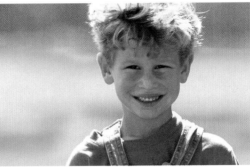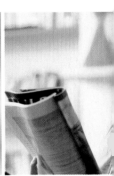

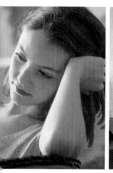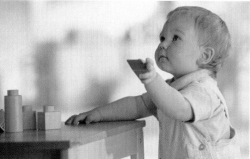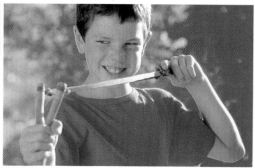

CHAPTER THREE
Behavioural and emotional problems 172

CHAPTER FOUR
Developmental problems and special needs 194

CHAPTER FIVE
Coping with emergencies 208

CHAPTER ONE

Maintaining your child's health

All parents want their child to be well and healthy, and it is natural to worry about your child's wellbeing. There are several steps you can take to help keep your child safe and well. Learning how to care for your child properly – from putting him to bed to ensuring his shoes fit – can help avoid illness and discomfort. Immunization can prevent many of the infectious diseases that afflicted children in the past.

Giving your child nutritious food will play a part in maintaining his health, and taking precautions against accidents will help keep him safe. Taking your child for routine health contacts will reassure you he is developing as he should or enable problems to be treated quickly. There are also ways to promote your child's development.

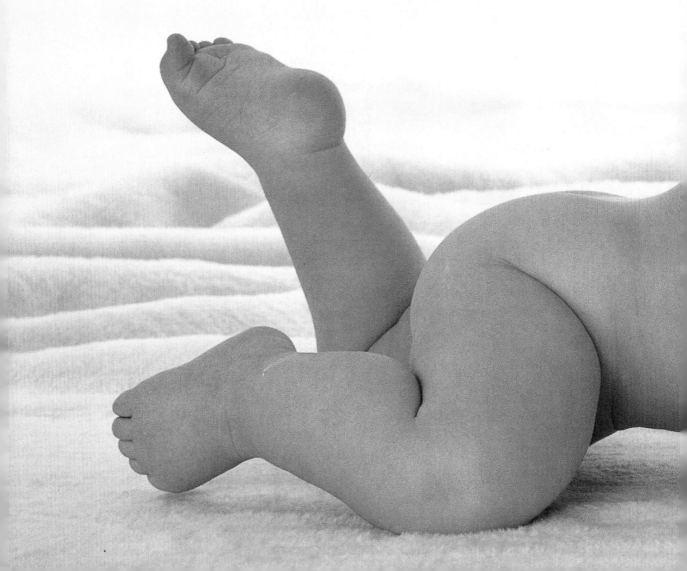

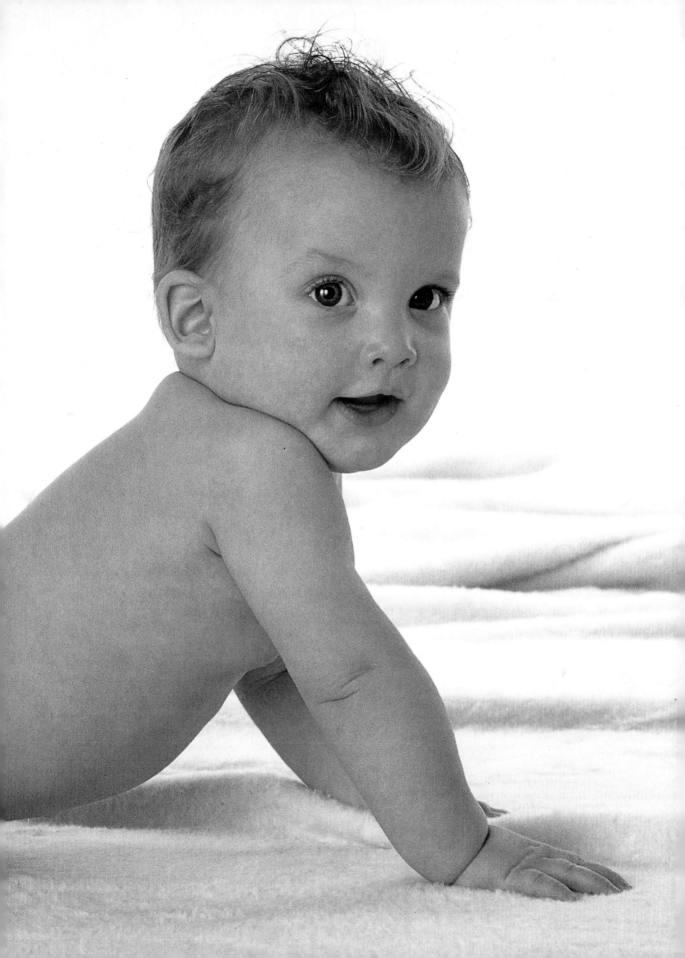

Your newborn baby

Immediately after birth your baby will be examined by the midwife or doctor to ensure that everything is well. Your baby's skin may look wrinkled, red or blotchy and her eyes may be puffy – this is normal in healthy babies.

Your newborn baby

All newborn babies vary considerably in terms of size, colour and shape. Very few look like the babies frequently seen in advertisements, who are usually weeks or months old.

The skin may be covered with vernix, a white protective substance, when your baby is born. This can be washed off or allowed to disappear. An overdue baby may have dry, flaky skin. Most babies get blotches, spots or rashes in the first few weeks. These are harmless and clear up without treatment. The skin may be mottled, or one part of the body may be pale and the other part red, due to an immature circulatory system. Birthmarks are common, but they are often temporary.

Before the umbilical cord is cut it is clamped and the remaining stump may be treated to prevent infection. The stump usually shrivels and falls off in about a week to 10 days, leaving behind the belly button. Normally, all you need to do is to keep the stump clean – using tap water – and dry. Inform the doctor or midwife if there is any bleeding or discharge.

The newborn's head

The head of a newborn baby is large in relation to her body. The head may also be elongated where it was squeezed or moulded through the birth canal during delivery. This temporary condition will disappear in a week or two. There may be a soft swelling, or caput, toward the back

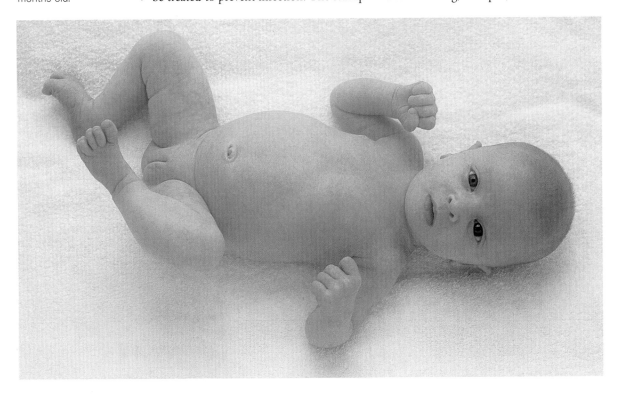

of the head due to pressure; it soon disappears. Some babies have a cystlike swelling on one or both sides of the head, known as a cephalhaematoma; it may take up to a few months to disappear.

The fontanelles are soft spots on your baby's head, where the scalp bones have not yet joined together. Although there is no bone, the spots are covered by a membrane and normally pulsate. There is no danger to the baby if they are handled in a normal manner. The back fontanelle closes in 6 to 8 weeks, but the larger front fontanelle closes over 18 months to 2 years. If the fontanelles are sunken or depressed, the baby may be dehydrated. A bulging fontanelle may be a sign of an illness such as meningitis – contact your doctor immediately.

Facial features

Most babies are born with blue-grey eyes, but the colour may change during the first six months. A baby can see from birth, but fully mature vision takes a few years to develop. A newborn's eyes may be puffy or have marks on the eyelids because of pressure from the birth; they will disappear. A young baby may sometimes appear to squint; if this happens a lot or after she is six months old, you should seek advice from your health visitor or doctor.

Babies often get sticky or watery eyes because of blocked tear ducts. Most ducts clear within a few months, but it may take up to a year. To clean the eyes, dip a piece of cotton wool in boiled water that has been allowed to cool, and wipe once from the inner corner outward. Massaging the lower lid from the middle to the inner corner and back can help to open the duct. If there is a pussy discharge or the eye becomes red, antibiotic eye drops may be needed.

New babies often have pads or blisters on the upper and lower lips from sucking; these will disappear. A white tongue or white patches in the mouth that do not rub off may be due to thrush (see p.152).

It is common for babies to have a blocked or stuffy nose. Do not use decongestant drops unless prescribed by your doctor, and then only for a few days. Prolonged use can make the condition worse. Raising the mattress a little and using saline nose drops can help.

A normal baby can hear sounds from birth. If there is a discharge from an ear, you should speak to your doctor. Some babies may be born with no hair, but it will grow over time. Others may have lots of hair, which usually falls out gradually over a few months. It will then regrow.

Irregular breathing

It is normal for a newborn baby to breathe irregularly, with about 40 to 60 breaths a minute. However, you should contact your doctor if your baby's lips or face turn pale or blue, or if her chest is drawn in as she breathes.

JAUNDICE

Most babies develop a yellowish discoloration of the skin and the whites of the eyes during the second to fourth day of life. This is physiological jaundice and is due to a temporary build-up of the pigment bilirubin. Bilirubin is formed during the breakdown of old red blood cells and is cleared by the liver. In new babies this process may not work well at first, but the jaundice usually clears in full-term babies at 7 days and in premature babies at 14 days. In breastfed babies the jaundice may last for two weeks or disappear and reappear after two to three weeks and persist for four months.

For some babies, however, jaundice may be a sign of a serious but treatable liver disease. Tests will need to be carried out and treatment started urgently if necessary.

You should contact your doctor if:
- The jaundice appears within 24 hours of birth
- It persists for more than two weeks
- Your baby has pale stools and dark urine.

The reproductive system

After birth, your baby's genitals will be carefully inspected to make sure there are no problems such as undescended testes. Even after reassurance, however, parents who are unfamiliar with a young baby may sometimes be alarmed by the appearance of their baby's genitals. In both boys and girls, these are often red and swollen immediately after birth and may seem large in relation to the size of the body. This is usually due to the effect of the hormones produced by the mother during pregnancy and is harmless.

BABIES IN SPECIAL CARE

About 1 in 10 babies will need to stay in a special care unit because they are very small, premature or seriously ill. Because he has no protective fat, and it is very important that a premature baby is kept warm, he will be placed in an incubator where the temperature can be adjusted as necessary.

Depending on how premature your baby is, it may be necessary to give him oxygen or artificial ventilation to help him breathe, and his heart rate, respiration and other body functions may be monitored continuously. Because he may be too weak to suck at first, a tube may be passed through his nose and into his stomach for breast milk or a formula. Breast milk is especially beneficial for premature babies and you will be encouraged to express your breast milk if you want to breastfeed.

Having a baby in special care can be distressing for parents, but you will be encouraged by the hospital staff to visit as often as you wish and to stroke his hand through portholes in the incubator until he is well enough for a cuddle.

Although the prognosis for babies born at less than 23 weeks is very poor, the overall survival of premature babies has improved significantly in industrialized countries.

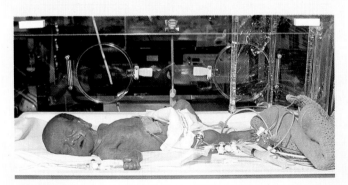

A girl may have a swollen clitoris and sometimes have a white or bloodstained discharge from the vagina. Again, this is usually due to hormones from the mother and the condition should clear up in a few days without treatment. If it persists, then you should contact your doctor.

In boys, the scrotum may be large and wrinkled, and there may be a hydrocele, a build-up of fluid around the testicles (see pp.160–161). The fluid will gradually be reabsorbed into the body over a few months.

As the baby develops in the womb, the testes develop in the abdomen in a male foetus, and descend into the scrotum shortly before birth. The doctor will check that the testes have descended. At birth, about 60 in 1,000 males have one or both of their testes undescended, although the rate is much higher in premature babies. The testes will be checked again at the routine six to eight week examination, and by the age of three months, they will have descended normally in many babies. Long-term problems, such as infertility or tumours, may arise if the testicles are left undescended; in this case, the baby should be referred to a surgeon before he is 18 months old.

Both boys and girls sometimes have swollen breasts, and there may be a milky discharge. These are due to the effects of the mother's hormones and should be left alone. The swelling will disappear without treatment over a few weeks.

The first stools

When a baby is born, the first stools will appear as a sticky, greenish black substance, known as meconium. If this is not passed within the first 48 hours, it could indicate that there is a problem in the digestive system, which must be investigated by the doctor.

Over the next few days, a baby's stools will change from greenish black to a greenish brown colour, then to a yellow or mustard colour. The stools are often runny in breastfed babies, but bottlefed babies usually have larger, firmer stools. The number of stools that are passed during the day will vary with each baby. As long as the stools are soft and a normal colour, there is no need to worry if your baby does not produce stools every day.

Passing urine

Most babies will pass urine within the first few hours after birth. The urine is normally light to dark yellow. Sometimes the nappy may be stained pink in the first week or two. This is due to the baby excreting urates, which are harmless salts of uric acid.

Blood in the urine is not normal in babies; at the first sign report it to your doctor. Other reasons to contact your doctor include if your baby strains or appears to be in pain when passing urine.

WHAT TO GET BEFORE THE BABY ARRIVES	
Basic items	**What to look for**
For feeding	If you're breastfeeding, you may wish to buy a breast pump to express the milk, as well as some plastic baby bottles to store breast milk in. To bottlefeed, you'll need several large baby bottles and a few small ones.
Clothing	Babies grow quickly. Start with items for up to three month olds, and buy new ones before your baby grows into them. Your baby will need six sleepers, front-opening outfits, cotton vests and bibs; two jumpers and pairs of socks or booties; a sunbonnet or a warm hat, coat and gloves.
For hygiene	Start off with six to eight dozen disposable nappies for the first week or two dozen cloth nappies, along with nappy pins and protective pants. You'll need a sturdy surface for changing nappies. You may wish to get a nappy carrier bag. For bathing, a few terry baby towels will do.
Large equipment	You'll need a cot, with blankets and sheets (see pp.18–19); a baby seat until the baby can sit up on her own (some convert into a car seat); and a pushchair. You may want an automatic swing, which many babies find soothing. Avoid using a walker – it can cause a severe accident.

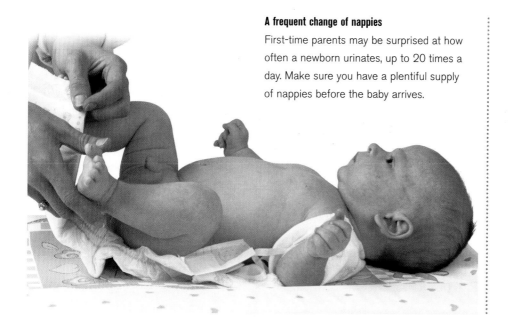

A frequent change of nappies

First-time parents may be surprised at how often a newborn urinates, up to 20 times a day. Make sure you have a plentiful supply of nappies before the baby arrives.

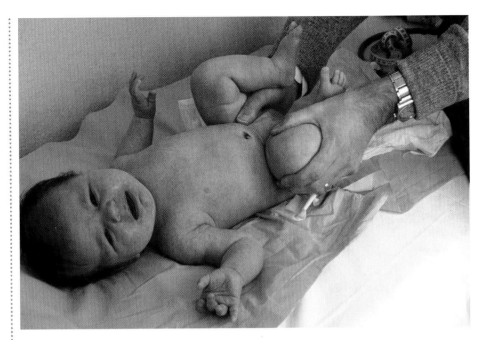

Testing a newborn baby
A newborn will undergo a variety of tests to make sure she is healthy. This includes manipulating the hips to check for a congential hip dislocation.

Legs and feet

Parents are often concerned about the shape and position of their baby's feet and legs at birth. Most problems are, however, common minor deformities and will correct themselves as the child grows, without any treatment being required.

WEIGHT

Newborns vary in size and weight. The average weight is 3.5 kg (7 lb 12 oz). Most healthy full-term babies weigh between 2.7 kg (5 lb 15 oz) and 4.3 kg (9 lb 8 oz) if they are boys and between 2.6 kg (5 lb 10 oz) and 4.1 kg (9 lb) if they are girls. A low birth weight baby is classified as being less than 2.5 kg (5 lb 8 oz). A very low birth weight is below 1.5 kg (3 lb 5 oz).

It is normal for babies to lose weight during the first few days, and some may lose up to 10 percent of their body weight in the first week. Birth weight is usually regained by the end of the second week. Most babies double their birth weight by four to five months, and treble their birth weight by one year.

Your baby's weight gain is a good guide to her overall progress and will be charted at the child health clinic on a growth chart. It is important not to get too anxious about your child's weight. Some babies will gain more weight some weeks than others, and in some weeks they may not gain any at all. This doesn't matter, as long as your baby is happy and active, looks well and gains weight over a period of weeks.

All babies will appear to have flat feet at birth. This is because the supporting arches in the feet are hidden by pads of fat and they don't fully develop until the child reaches the age of about six. The toes may turn inward so that the child looks pigeon-toed. This is a common problem, which will usually right itself by the time the child reaches 18 months old.

Sometimes, one foot or both feet may be twisted downward and inward, or twisted upward. This is known as club foot, or talipes (see p.131). It can occur if pressure was exerted on the foot while the child was in the womb. In most cases, talipes will correct itself without treatment – only in severe cases will treatment be required.

Your baby's legs and hips will be checked at birth and again during further routine checks for a congenital dislocation of the hip (see p.129), or clicky hip. This can cause a limp if it is not treated. In some cases, the joints may be unstable, rather than dislocated.

Reflexes

All newborn babies have certain reflexes. A reflex is an automatic response or reaction to a particular stimulus and is designed to protect the baby or help it to survive. Some of these reflexes disappear quite quickly, others last a few months.

After your baby is born, the doctor may check for these reflexes and will do so again at the routine six to eight week check. Abnormal or absent reflexes, or the persistence of certain reflexes after the time they should have disappeared, could be a sign of neurological damage.

Types of reflex

● Rooting reflex: if you gently stroke your baby's cheek, she will turn her head in the direction of the side touched for something to suck. She will also open her mouth. This action helps her search for the nipple when breastfeeding.
● Sucking reflex: this is crucial to your baby's survival. When a nipple, teat or even your finger is placed in your baby's mouth, she will place her lips around it, lower her tongue and begin to suck. This reflex is present before birth – an ultrasound test may show your baby sucking her thumb.
● Grasp reflex: if you place your finger in your baby's hand, she will grasp it tightly. This grasp is so strong in the first few days after birth that if she grasped the finger with both hands, she could hold her own weight momentarily – but do not try to make her do this yourself.
● Babinski reflex: if you stroke the sole of her foot, her toes will curl.
● Startle, or Moro, reflex: if your baby is scared or startled by a sudden noise or movement, she will react by flinging her legs and arms wide, with fingers extended, and arching her back. She will then bring her arms and legs together and may cry. This reflex gives a good indication of the condition of the baby's muscle tone and her nervous system.
● Walking or stepping reflex: if you hold your newborn baby under the arms in an upright position and let her feet touch a flat surface, she will lift her leg up, place one foot in front of the other and "walk". This reflex disappears after five to six weeks and she then has to learn to walk.
● Blinking reflex: a baby will blink at bright light or sudden movement.

SEE ALSO

Meningitis	66–67
Birthmarks	104
Flat feet	130
Problems of the testes	160–161

Typical reflexes
A healthy newborn baby will have several automatic reflexes, some of which will disappear with time.

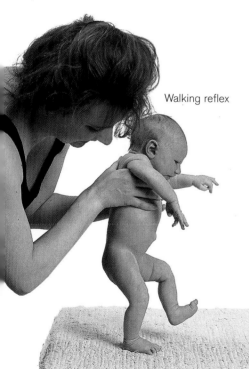
Walking reflex

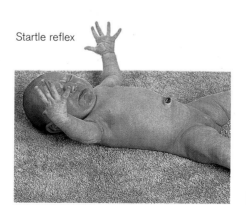
Startle reflex

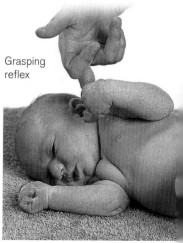
Grasping reflex

Bathing your baby and helping him to sleep

New parents are often apprehensive about caring for a new baby – how do they bath him, successfully help him fall asleep or understand why he is crying?

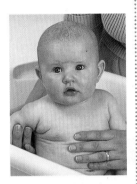

The cardinal safety rule
Never leave a baby or toddler alone in the bath, even for a moment. He can drown in as little as 8 cm (3 in) of water.

With a little confidence, patience and practice, caring for your child will soon become second nature. You may find that learning why your baby is crying is the most difficult part of getting him to stop (see box, below). Although many babies protest vigorously at first when it comes to bathing, they soon learn to enjoy the experience, and getting your baby quietly to sleep may require only a little perseverance on your part.

A CRYING BABY

Your baby may cry a lot in the early weeks because crying is the only way he has of communicating with you. By crying, your baby is telling you one of a number of things. You will soon begin to recognize his different cries and respond accordingly. Here are the most likely reasons that a baby is crying:

- Hunger – if you think your baby is hungry, offer him your breast or a bottle. Most babies need feeding on demand during the early weeks of life.
- Check that your baby is not too hot or cold – the best area on a baby to judge this is the abdomen.
- Check for any discomfort – his clothes may be too tight or twisted or he may have a wet or soiled nappy.
- Your baby may simply need reassurance – give him a cuddle.
- He may be bored, tired or overstimulated.
- Some babies cry if they are teething or if they are ill – colic is a common cause of crying in babies under three months old.

Research has shown that mothers who respond quickly to their baby's cries have babies who are more contented and secure as a result. Follow your instinct when your baby is crying, and don't worry about spoiling him if he wants frequent nursing.

Some babies cry more than others, but if you feel that your baby cries excessively or he never stops crying, no matter what you do, consult your doctor or health visitor.

Bathtime

There is no need to bath a baby for a week or two after birth, and you may be advised not to until the stump of the umbilical cord falls off. Even then, two to three baths a week is plenty. In between, clean his face, behind his ears, the skin folds of his neck and armpits and his entire nappy area daily – this is known as topping and tailing. Clean his face and hands and nappy area as necessary.

There is no need to buy a special baby bath unless you want to. A sink may be adequate until your baby can sit in the big bath. Before starting, make sure you have everything you need to hand and that the room is warm and free from draughts. Put the water in the bowl or bath, and check the water with the inside of your wrist or your elbow to make sure it is comfortably warm, not too hot. Use a mild baby soap or mild baby bath solution. Wash your baby's face with a separate bowl of plain warm water and cotton wool before giving him his bath.

Sleeping

For the first few weeks, your newborn will sleep and wake at random. The number of hours a new baby sleeps for varies; some sleep for 14 hours or more, others for less.

When feeding your baby during the night talk to him quietly and keep the light dim so that he gradually begins to recognize that night-time is for sleeping.

Rather than breastfeeding your baby to sleep, put him into his cot while he is awake so that he learns to fall asleep in it. Babies who are used to being breastfed to sleep often refuse to settle down without being breastfed if they wake during the night. Some babies also need to cry themselves to sleep. Always remember to put your baby to sleep on his back.

How soon you settle your baby into a regular sleep routine is up to you. Some parents prefer to put their baby to bed early in the evening, others put their baby to sleep in his cot when they go to bed.

SEE ALSO

Sudden infant death syndrome	18–19
Colic	93
Sleeping problems	184–185

Washing your baby's hair

Wrap your baby in a towel and tuck him under your arm. Support his back with your arm and his head with your hand; hold him face up. With your free hand, wash and rinse his hair. You don't need shampoo at first. Towel dry his hair.

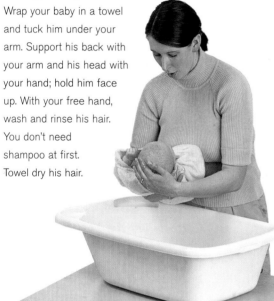

Lowering your baby into the bath

Unwrap your baby, remove his nappy and clean any soiling. Place one arm behind your baby's back, with your hand gripping the arm furthest away from you. With your other hand, support his legs and buttocks and lower him into the bath, bottom first.

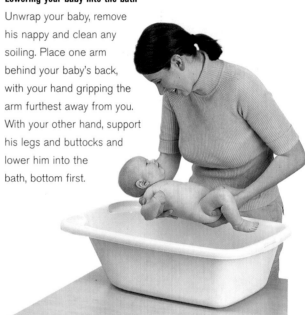

Bathing your baby

While supporting his head and shoulders, wash his body. To wash his back, sit him up and rest his chest on your arm. Help him enjoy his bath by talking to him and smiling; gently splash some water.

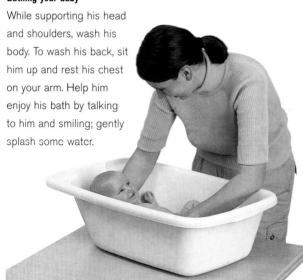

Drying your baby

Keeping one hand firmly behind his shoulder, slide the other hand under his buttocks and lift him out of the bath. Dry your baby carefully, especially in the folds of the skin.

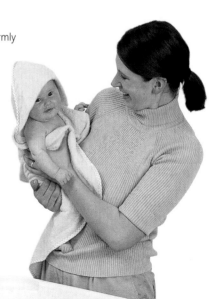

Sudden infant death syndrome

The unexpected death of a baby, for which there is no identifiable explanation – even after a post mortem – is called sudden infant death syndrome (SIDS), or cot death.

The feet to foot position

By placing your baby with her feet to the foot of the cot, you'll prevent her from wriggling down underneath the bedclothes in the cot.

The cause of cot death is still not understood; in recent years, however, the death rate has fallen after parents were advised to place their babies on their backs when lying them down to sleep. Despite the common name cot death, the syndrome can occur anywhere – in the pram, in a car or in someone's arms.

You can reduce the risk of cot death by getting medical advice if your baby is unwell. You should seek urgent medical attention if she has a high temperature,

has breathing difficulties or turns blue, is less responsive than usual, has glazed eye or cannot focus them, you cannot wake her or she has a febrile seizure.

While no one can guarantee the prevention of cot death, it is still rare, so don't let worrying about it spoil your enjoyment of your baby. A number of factors have been identified as putting a baby at risk (see box, opposite), and it is thought that a combination of factors may be responsible for a death, rather

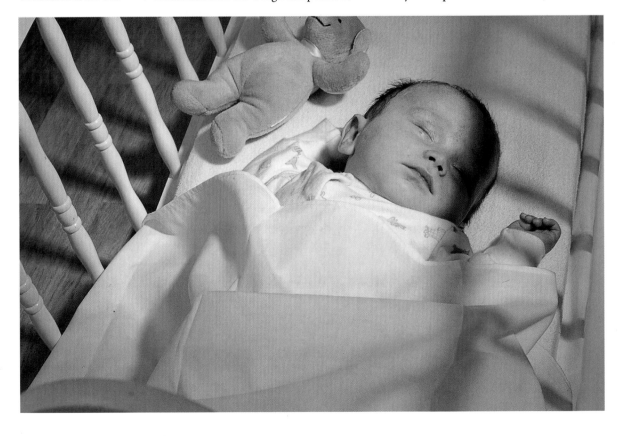

WHO'S AT RISK

While cot death can happen to any baby, it is known that some babies are at greater risk. These include:

- Premature, low birth weight babies
- Babies whose parents are smokers
- Twins
- Babies of young, poor mothers
- Boy babies are more at risk than girls, although the reason is not known
- Babies of mothers under 25 years who already have other children.

than a single cause. There are ways in which you can reduce the risk.

(If you have serious concerns about cot death – if you have perhaps lost a previous baby in this way – ask your doctor for information on alarms that warn when a baby stops breathing, and do all you can to eliminate any risk factors.)

Putting your baby to bed

Always put your baby to sleep on her back unless there are medical reasons not to do so. Research has found that this is much safer than placing a baby on her tummy. As your baby gets older she will roll or move into the position most comfortable for her. This is little cause for concern, because there is less risk if she sleeps on her side than on her tummy, and the risk of cot death in babies over six months old is extremely low.

Place your baby to sleep on her back in the feet to foot position, with her feet touching the foot of the cot. This prevents her from moving down, possibly covering her head with the bedclothes. You should keep your baby's head uncovered while she is in the cot and tuck her in with a sheet and blanket. Don't give a baby under the age of one a pillow.

Avoid overheating the room, and don't let your baby become too hot. Feeling her tummy is a good way to judge how warm she is. You should keep the bedroom at a temperature that is comfortable, about 16–20°C (60–68°F); keep a thermometer in the room. Don't use duvets, quilts, cot bumpers, baby nests or sheepskins – they may cause the baby to overheat.

Other ways to reduce risks

You should also avoid overheating your baby in other environments. Take off her hat and extra clothing as soon as you come indoors or enter a warm car, bus or train, even if it means waking her.

Research has found that smoking may account for more than half of all cases of cot death. Both parents should stop smoking in pregnancy. Don't let anyone smoke in the same room as your baby or let anyone have contact with your baby if they have smoked in the last 30 to 60 minutes – smoke will still be present in the expired air. Establish your baby's sleeping place as a smoke-free zone.

Don't let your baby sleep while propped up on a cushion on a sofa or armchair. Although parents may enjoy taking their baby into bed with them for feeding or comfort, it is preferable to place your baby in the cot to sleep. Parents who smoke and share a bed with their baby may increase the risk of cot death. If you wish your baby to sleep in your bed, don't smoke, drink alcohol or take sleeping pills or illegal drugs before going to sleep. Your baby can sleep in the same room for as long as you want.

Studies have found that immunization is associated with a decreased risk of cot death – not an increased risk, as some parents have feared. Fears about flying seem to also be unfounded; flying is believed to be safe for healthy babies.

Immunization

Certain potentially dangerous diseases can be prevented by introducing specific agents into the body to trigger the immune system into action artificially – this is known as immunization, or vaccination.

A vaccine may contain part of a bacteria or virus with its poison rendered harmless, or a weakened form of the live bacteria or virus. It stimulates the body to make antibodies without incurring the major risks of the disease. If your child then comes into contact with the disease, the antibodies protect him against the infection.

All countries have immunization programmes to protect against major diseases, but the schedule may vary. They include protection against diphtheria, pertussis (whooping cough), tetanus, polio, measles, mumps, rubella (German measles), tuberculosis (TB) and a strain of *Haemophilus influenzae* type B (Hib). Some countries offer routine protection against group C meningococcal disease, varicella (chickenpox) and hepatitis B. Other immunizations are available against

influenza and pneumococcus if your child needs protection against these diseases.

It is important to protect a child against the major diseases, which may have serious complications or result in death. Some diseases are rarely seen in industrialized countries but are rife in other countries. If immunization declines, these diseases may be introduced by travellers from areas where they still exist, and unimmunized children will be at risk. There will also be a rise in infectious diseases, such as measles, mumps and whooping cough, if not enough children are immunized against them.

Vaccine safety and side effects

After immunization, you can give your child a dose of paracetamol. In many cases, this will prevent him getting a fever. (Never give a child under 12 years old aspirin; see p.63.) Some parents are concerned about the safety of a vaccine. Vaccines can only be licensed for use after rigorous testing for their effectiveness and safety. There may be side effects, but most of them are not serious. These include:
● Diphtheria, pertussis and tetanus (DPT) vaccine may cause irritability, a fever or a lump and inflammation at the injection site. Rarely, fits may occur; in 1 in every 110,000 injections, there may be inflammation of the brain. In a rare case when a child has a severe reaction, your doctor may advice that no further doses of the pertussis component are given.

Providing immunity
Although reactions to vaccines can occur, these are generally mild, and complications from the diseases themselves are far greater than those caused by the vaccine.

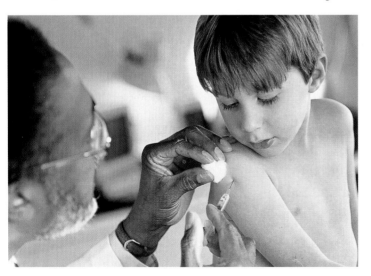

- About 1 in 10 children experiences redness and a small swelling where the Hib vaccine is injected; this will disappear.
- For about every 2 million doses of polio vaccine given, one child will get the disease. After your baby is given the vaccine, it is excreted in the stools for six weeks. If a person who has not been immunized against polio changes the baby's nappy, she must thoroughly wash her hands afterward.
- The measles part of a measles, mumps and rubella (MMR) vaccine may cause illness, and a rash may appear 7 to 14 days later. Rarely, the mumps part may cause a mild form of mumps three weeks after the injection. The rubella part may cause a rash. One in 3,000 children has a fit. One child in a million will have encephalitis, but the rate is the same without the vaccine. One child in 5,000 will have encephalitis after measles disease.

When to avoid vaccination

Sometimes an immunization may need to be postponed, and some children should not receive certain vaccines. Tell your doctor if your child has an acute illness with a fever, an allergy to eggs, a bad reaction to a previous immunization or has had fits or convulsions in the past. Also tell him if your child, you or anyone else in the family is being treated for a malignant disease with chemotherapy or radiotherapy, is on high doses of steroids or has HIV or AIDS (see p.73).

If your child has a minor illness, such as a cold, or is on antibiotics but is otherwise well, he can be immunized. Children with asthma or eczema can also be immunized. Children who are allergic to eggs can usually be given MMR, but consult your doctor. Premature babies should start their routine immunizations two months after birth, the same age as other babies.

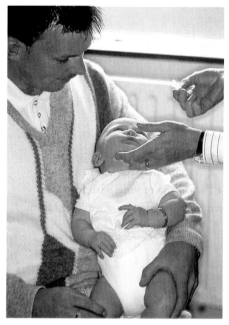

Vaccinating against polio
Not all immunization is provided with a needle and syringe – vaccination against polio is given by placing drops in the mouth.

SEE ALSO

Infectious diseases	**60–61**
Meningitis	**66–67**
Encephalitis	**166**
Febrile convulsions	**167**

IMMUNIZATION SCHEDULE UP TO AGE 13

At 2, 3 and 4 months	12–15 months	3–5 years (usually before the child starts school)	10–13 years

Polio
  By mouth
 	
Diphtheria
Pertussis
Tetanus (DPT)
  One injection
 	
Hib
  May be given
  on its own or
  added to the
  DPT injection
 	
Group C
meningococcal
disease
  By injection
	Measles
	Mumps
	Rubella (MMR)
	  One injection
		Measles
		Mumps
		Rubella (MMR)
		  One injection
		
		Diphtheria
		Tetanus
		  One injection
		
		Polio
		  By mouth
			Tuberculosis
			  Skin test;
			  injection
			  (BCG) if
			  needed.
			  (May be given
			  after birth
			  if there is
			  exposure to
			  the disease.)
			
			Note: DPT
			(see far left)
			may also
			be given
			to 15–16
			year olds

Milestones: newborn to age 2

All children grow and develop at their own pace, but the majority of healthy children will reach what are called developmental milestones by a certain age.

A busy year

During your child's first year, he will learn how to sit, crawl, grasp items, stand, and he may even begin to walk and talk.

There is an enormous range in the normal heights and weights of children. It is only when children fall outside this range that there may be a reason for concern. Children grow most rapidly during their first two years. Their growth will then slow down, and they will experience a much longer period of steady but slower growth before they have a short period of rapid growth during puberty (see pp.28–29).

For the first five years of your child's life, her head circumference, weight and height will be monitored at a health clinic, using a centile chart. This chart is essentially a mathematical guide to how children normally grow. There are different charts for boys and girls, because boys are usually taller and heavier than girls.

The curved centile lines on the charts roughly show the growth patterns of normal babies. There is a middle line that represents the national average – 50 percent of children have measurements that fall below this line and 50 percent of children have them above it. It doesn't matter where your baby starts on the chart, whether it is above or below the middle centile line or if she crosses one or two of the other centile lines, as long as she is otherwise healthy.

When to see a doctor

You should make an appointment for your child to see a doctor if her height falls below what is known as the 0.4th centile or above the 99.6th centile. You should also make an appointment if there is a change from her normal pattern – for example, if your child's weight begins to drop rapidly.

There are several factors that can affect the normal growth of a child. These include heredity, nutritional disorders, such as untreated coeliac disease (see p.99), and chronic illnesses. Rarely, short stature may be caused by a an endocrine or chromosomal disorder, and excessive growth by a hormonal abnormality or certain rare syndromes. If you are worried that your child does not appear to be growing normally, you should ask your doctor to refer you to a paediatrician for an assessment.

DEVELOPMENTAL WATCH

Check with your health visitor or doctor if:

- You are worried about your baby's hearing at any time.
- By the time your baby reaches three months, she is not smiling or has poor head control.
- At six months your baby does not roll or grasp or transfer objects.
- Your baby cannot sit at nine months.
- She cannot crawl, pick up tiny objects such as crumbs with her finger and thumb, does not make sounds such as "mamma" or "dada" by 12 months.
- Your baby cannot walk without support, understand simple sentences or does not jabber or say single words at 18 months.

Developmental milestones

In general, your baby will double her birth weight during the first five to six months of life. By 12 months, she will triple it and be 25–30 cm (10–12 in) longer (see chart below).

If your baby was premature, assess her development from the expected date of delivery, not her actual date of birth. For example, a nine month old baby born three months premature has the developmental level of a six month old.

SEE ALSO

Milestones: ages 2–6   **24–25**

Milestones: ages 6–12   **26–27**

Identifying a child with developmental delay   **196–197**

DEVELOPMENTAL MILESTONES

Age	What child can do
6 weeks–3 months	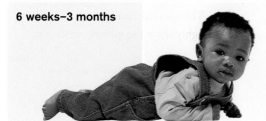 • By the time your baby is six weeks old, she will turn her head and eyes toward light, begin to watch her mother's face and respond to speech. If whimpering, she will quieten to the sound of her mother's voice and smile. She can hold her head up for a short period without wobbling. • By three months, your baby will grasp an object put in her hand, smile spontaneously, coo, kick and hold her head up steadily.
3–6 months	• If you take her hands, she might try to pull herself up into a sitting position. • Your baby can roll from her stomach on to her back. • She may reach out to grasp an object, and she can bring her hands together on her own. • She recognizes familiar people and smiles at other babies.
6–9 months	• Now she can grasp objects such as a rattle in one hand and transfer this to the other hand. • Your baby can roll over and back, sit without support for longer periods and bear her weight on her feet when supported. • Your baby can hold a bottle, finger feed and chew lumps. • She will imitate a cough, laugh and squeal and start to make different sounds such as "dada".
9–12 months	• Your baby will crawl or bottom shuffle, pull herself up to stand, cruise around furniture or even walk. • She understands the meaning of "no", can claps hands, may say several words and may respond to commands.
1–2 years	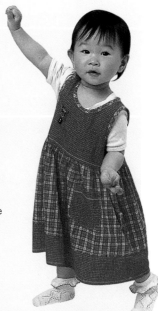• Your child will learn to walk and climb and will be getting into everything. She can sit and ride on a truck. • She will use 6 to 20 or more single words and start to join words together to form phrases. • Your baby will enjoy copying household tasks such as dusting, and she will understand simple requests such as to fetch your shoes. • She will be able to hold a spoon and take it to her mouth, and she will start scribbling. • Your baby may also start to throw temper tantrums (see pp.178–179).

Milestones: ages 2–6

During this period your child's physical growth will slow down, although he will continue to grow steadily. At the same time, his coordination and his intellectual, emotional and social skills will rapidly improve.

By the age of two, your child's fontanelles (soft spots on top of head) will have fused together. Between the first and second years, he will gain 2–3 kg (4–7 lb) in weight, and his height will be about half of his adult height. On average, your child will gain 2 kg (4 lb) each year, with a minimum growth of 6 cm (2½ in) a year. If your child grows less than 5 cm (2 in) per year between the ages of two and five, he should be seen by a doctor. Remember, boys are often taller and heavier than girls of the same age.

Your child's intellectual, social and emotional development will also advance. By the time your child is six, he will be able to reason with you in a way that he couldn't as a two-year-old toddler.

At first, when your child begins to walk and talk, he may seem clumsy or it may be difficult for anyone outside the family to understand what he is saying – this is

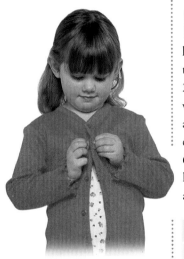

Hand skills

By three years of age, your child's confidence will increase. She may begin to try tasks that require coordination such as doing up the buttons on a cardigan.

DEVELOPMENTAL MILESTONES

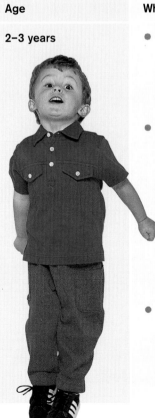

Age	What child can do
2–3 years	• The two-year-old child is egocentric; that is, he is the centre of his own world. He cannot understand the concept of sharing. Giving his toys to another child is likely to provoke howls of rage. The two year old watches other children play and plays near them, but not with them. By the age of three, he plays with other children and understands sharing.
	• From the age of two he may start to indicate his toilet needs, and by the age of three he is usually dry during the day. Boys are usually ready to start toilet training at two and a half years, but girls will have started earlier.
	• At two years old your child will be getting up and down stairs by holding on and will begin to jump with both feet. He knows five body parts, uses about 50 words and he may put 2 or 3 words together in a simple sentence. He understands longer instructions such as "put the cup on the table" and asks for food and drink. He can do simple puzzles, point to items in pictures, turn a door knob, unscrew a lid and build a tower of five bricks.
	• By two and a half years, your child can jump with both feet; walk up and down stairs without help; and kick a ball without falling. He talks in short sentences and knows one colour. He uses pronouns such as me, you and I, has started to ask questions, and understands simple short stories and conversations.

normal. There are times, however, when your child should be checked by your doctor or health visitor. These include if you feel your child is abnormally clumsy or falls over too much, you are concerned about his hearing, he is not putting two or three words together by the time he reaches 27 months, he cannot be understood by strangers at the age of four, he does not respond to people outside the family or he is not normally dry during the day by the age of three.

SEE ALSO
Routine health contacts   **30–31**
Speech and language problems   **200–201**
Hearing difficulties   **202–203**

DEVELOPMENTAL MILESTONES

Age	What child can do
3–4 years	• The three year old can carry on a simple conversation and will ask questions incessantly – where, what and why? He will carry on a monologue, and he knows nursery rhymes and may sing them. He understands more complicated sentences such as "go upstairs to the bathroom and fetch the soap". He begins to dress and undress himself with help. • He can build a tower of nine bricks, knows some colours and may count to 10. He draws circles and copies a cross if shown how to. He eats with a fork and spoon. He can ride a pedal cycle and stand briefly on one foot; he enjoys pretend play.

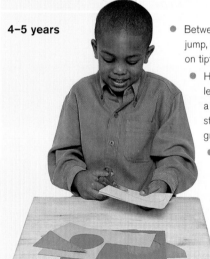

Age	What child can do
4–5 years	• Between the ages of four and five, your child can hop, jump, skip, ride a tricycle or bicycle with stabilizers, run on tiptoe and climb. • He has a mature pencil grasp and can copy basic letters, and he can draw a square and a person with a round head and stick limbs. He loves listening to stories and enjoys simple jokes. His speech is grammatically correct, but he may invent words. • He enjoys playing with other children and can take turns. He can dress and undress except for difficult fastenings. He appreciates past, present and future time, and can give his full name, age and usually his address. • Bed-wetting is considered normal up to the age of five.
5–6 years	• At five years, he begins to reason and to make comparisons, and he understands that we all have our own thoughts. By the time he is six years old, he can divide items into simple categories. • He may start mimicking the movements and voices of others around him. He can learn physical activities such as how to swim or skate. • Your child's drawings will become busier at five years old. By six years of age, your child may start to line up his drawing with the edge of the paper.

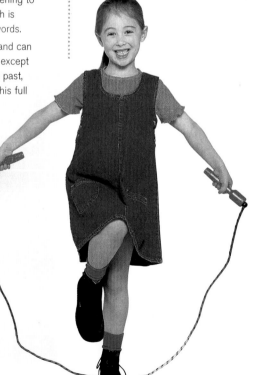

Milestones: ages 6–12

These years can be the happiest ones for a child and her family. The relationship between you and your child will become more companionable, and you may soon see glimpses of the adult that your child will become.

DEVELOPMENTAL MILESTONES

Age	Physical	Social
6–9 years	• A child of six is two-thirds the height she will be as an adult, and her brain ninetenths of its eventual size. Her chubbiness will disappear, and her legs will look longer in relation to the rest of her body. • A common characteristic of the six to eight year old is the child's gappy smile as the milk teeth fall out. They are quickly replaced by the child's permanent teeth. • There is usually a growth spurt around the age of seven. In boys, there is a perceptible broadening of the shoulders; in girls, a slight rounding of the hips. • Physical coordination improves markedly during this period – most children are able to ride a bicycle and kick and catch balls. Fine motor skills also improve – your child should be able to fasten buttons and tie shoe laces. Any problems associated with coordination should now be identified.	• She becomes more discerning about who she spends her time with and will choose friends with whom she has common interests. The friendships formed at this stage often last for life. • A child in this age group is usually sociable and enjoys organizations and clubs such as the Cubs or Brownies. She may experiment with other activities, but these may be short-term enthusiasms. • By the age of nine, she should be self sufficient and can entertain herself at times. 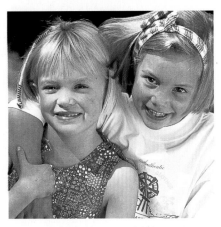
10–12 years	• The child is on the brink of puberty and should be told about the changes to expect. • The first sign of puberty in boys is the enlargement of the testes, followed by the growth of the penis and a rapid increase in height. Pubic hair and armpit hair appear later, and the voice begins to break. • The initial sign of puberty in girls is gradual swelling of the breasts and growth acceleration. If your daughter's periods start early, they will be erratic and slight in volume, and the blood may be watery. • Your child will now have all of her permanent teeth except her wisdom teeth – these normally appear in the mid to late teens.	• At this preteen stage, a child begins to demonstrate a desire to get on with being an adult and do things that older people do. • This is the age when experimentation with smoking and drinking may start. • Allow your child to make short trips away from home on her own, but make sure she knows how to use a public telephone and can read a bus or train timetable.

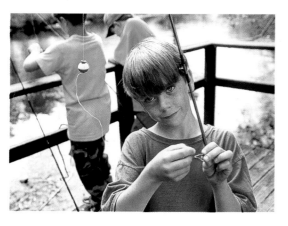

Becoming independent

As children enter their preteen years, they will become more selective when making friends and will want to choose the activities that they participate in. Don't be surprised if they wish to spend less time at home and more time with their friends.

SEE ALSO

Milestones: newborn
to age 2   22–23
Milestones: ages 2–6   24–25
Reaching puberty   28–29

DEVELOPMENTAL MILESTONES

Age	Intellectual	Emotional
6–9 years	• The school curriculum becomes more formalized because literacy and numeracy skills become a priority. • A six year old can usually read picture books with short, simple text; however, she may be so busy concentrating on identifying letters and words that she is not able to follow the story. • You should still read to her regularly so that she does not lose the pleasure of books at a point when reading may be a struggle. You can encourage her to read other forms of writing, including signs, programmes, posters and newspapers. • By the time your child is nine years old, she should be reading and enjoying a variety of books appropriate for her age. • Her handwriting should be fairly neat and legible, but spelling mistakes are common. • In mathematics she will progress from simple addition and subtraction to complicated mental arithmetic, multiplication and division.	• Although your child now has a life away from home, you remain her main reference point and she still requires lots of cuddling and reassurance on the occasions when things go wrong. • A child over the age of seven does not use temper tantrums to get her own way. She is more subtle in negotiating with her parents – but physical fights between brothers and sisters are still normal. 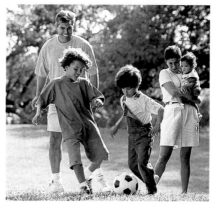
10–12 years	• This stage is marked by the important transition from primary to secondary education. Your child will have to cope with a much wider curriculum. • By now your child should be reading fluently, and the more advanced child can cope with suitable adult reading. • You should notice that your child has developed a clear, cursive handwriting style. • Your child's approach to learning becomes more analytical, and she should be able to understand another person's point of view.	• Despite physical signs of imminent sexual maturity, the sexes tend not to mix. In fact, there is often a great deal of antipathy between boys and girls at this age and most friends tend to be of the same sex. • This is the time when girls, in particular, may develop an intense crush on a pop star or film star. This "first love" can be intense and is one way in which the child can practise for future serious relationships outside the family.

Reaching puberty

Your child will grow in what seems like no time at all, and from six years of age through his preteen years, you'll notice changes that affect him not only physically but also emotionally and intellectually.

As your child becomes a preteenager, especially in the case of a girl, you'll become aware of the beginnings of change in body shape and growth. If you have a daughter she may start her periods, although only 10 percent of girls will do so before the age of 12. She will begin to put on weight due to the production of the hormone oestrogen, often doubling her weight by the time she is 18 years old.

Boys develop later, between the ages of 12 and 16; however, some boys develop pubic hair and facial "shadows" before they reach their teens. Your son's bones and muscles will increase in size when he begins making the hormone testosterone. Growth spurts will occur earlier in girls than in boys, making them temporarily taller and heavier.

Stages of puberty in a girl
The first signs will be her nipples enlarging and the appearance of breast buds, and she'll quickly gain in height and weight. Pubic hair will then begin to appear, but sometimes this may occur at an earlier stage. At the period of maximum growth, there is early breast development. About a year later her periods will start.

Emotional development

During these years, a child's emotional growth is important. It is a time when the process of separation from parents and development of independence take place. This does not happen in a smooth line going on and progressing toward adulthood, but in a jerky, spasmodic manner, with two steps toward maturity and one step back. You shouldn't be surprised if your child changes in his needs and attitude toward you from day to day – this is normal.

There will be times, even with older children, when he will need to be the baby and want a cuddle, although the next day he will be stretching his boundaries again and testing you to see how much you will allow. You should never refuse your child the security he needs or automatically refuse him independent acts because he was immature the day before. If you allow your child to express the emotions he feels at the time, he'll develop in a natural, well-rounded way.

Speech and vocabulary

As peers become important in your child's life, you may find that he emulates his friends' speech patterns and pronunciation, so for a while your normally

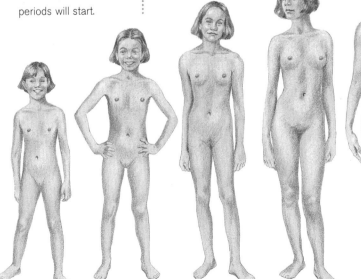

clear-speaking child may mumble or develop a lisp or another affectation. This is part of the bonding process children go through with their friends and, although you may find it irritating, it's best not to comment – it will soon pass.

Your child's vocabulary will increase dramatically throughout these years, and you should foster this by making time to listen carefully. You can discuss things in which he has an interest and allow time to talk about the books and television programmes you both enjoy.

Inevitably, at some stage, particular words or phrases you may wish that your child had not acquired will creep into his vocabulary. Strong swear words are often part of power play in the playground and, even if your child never hears you swear, he will learn the words from the outside world. Without lecturing, make it clear you do not want to hear these words. Learning what is appropriate is part of growing up, and it takes most children a while to grasp the concept of what is socially acceptable. If the language is racist or otherwise totally repugnant, it is worth approaching his school because they should be reinforcing your teaching why such speech is offensive.

Powers of persuasion

As your child gets older, he will grow intellectually, which means that he'll also learn how to become manipulative. It may take a harmless form, such as persuading you to let him stay at a friend's house for the weekend, and can have positive aspects in his friendships and in a future career. Equally, this trait may be used to his advantage in a way that you won't like.

For example, your child may say he is ill when he is not, he may not respond to you the first time you call him or he may insist he needs the volume of the television turned up to hear it.

Knowing when a complaint is real or not can be difficult. You should check with his teacher to see if she has noticed any problems with your child. Try to find out why he doesn't want to go to school. He may be worried about bullying or have a fear of failing (see pp.186–187). It is worth considering that although a sudden onset of deafness may be feigned, it may be that your child has a sinus problem or blocked ears are affecting his hearing. Depending on the situation, you may need to arrange for a consultation with your doctor.

Complaints about headaches (see p.166) should not automatically be attributed to his making it up, or to a lack of sleep, watching too much television or playing too many computer games. He may have a migraine, or he may have developed a vision problem or need a new prescription for his glasses. You should arrange for a sight test to be on the safe side.

SEE ALSO
Speech and language
problems   **200–201**
Hearing difficulties   **202–203**
Visual problems   **204–205**

Stages of puberty in a boy

The first sign of puberty is enlarged testes; the penis will begin to grow longer, and there will be a sharp increase in height. Pubic hair and hair under the armpits will appear, and his voice will break. When facial hair starts to grow, the young man will almost be his adult height. He'll reach physical and sexual maturity at 18 to 21 years of age.

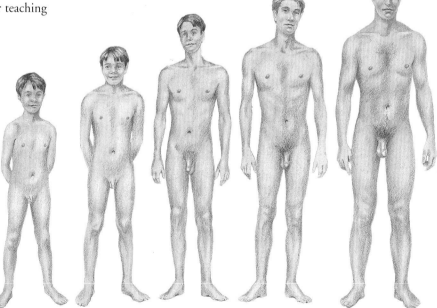

Routine health contacts

Your health visitor and doctor will help monitor your baby's overall progress and help you with any problems you encounter. To this end, you should take your child to the child health clinic or doctor's surgery at certain stages.

Routine contacts are made with all children at different ages from birth until they are five years old. At these contacts, you will have the opportunity to discuss with the doctor or health visitor any concerns you have and issues such as feeding, safety, immunization and behaviour. They will also monitor your child's development, and at set ages they will check for particular developmental or medical problems. They can also advise you what is reasonable for you to expect your child to be doing over the next weeks and months. These contacts may take place in the child health clinic, the doctor's surgery or at home.

The chart (opposite) outlines the minimum content of each contact. At most ages there will not be a physical examination, but the health visitor will discuss with you how your child is developing and will be ready to answer any questions that you have. The health visitor will assess whether your child's development is within the normal range in the spheres of speech and language, gross motor skills, such as crawling and walking, fine motor skills – how she uses her fingers and hands – and behaviour.

Some problems may go unnoticed by you, so it is important that you make use of these opportunities. Congenital heart disease, dislocation of the hips, eye problems such as squint, undescended testes and hearing problems may not be picked up unless they are deliberately sought. If you feel something is wrong, don't be afraid to ask. You are usually the best judge of your child's welfare.

Hearing screening

In an increasing number of areas, a baby's hearing is tested within a few days or weeks of birth. This tends to be done mainly in babies who were born prematurely or have been unwell, or where there is a close family history of early onset hearing impairment.

Many areas carry out a hearing screening test when a baby is between six and nine months old. It requires two trained people and a cooperative child. A baby may fail the test because she is tired or has a cold. A repeat test will be given and, if she fails again, she will be referred to a specialist. This test can be misleading and children with reduced hearing may appear to pass the test, so it is important to tell your health visitor if you have concerns about your child's hearing.

Measuring your baby's head
To check that she is developing normally, the circumference of your baby's head will be measured at six to eight weeks.

ROUTINE CONTACTS

Age	What will be monitored
Before your baby leaves hospital (usually by the doctor)	• General physical examination • Check for congenital dislocation of the hips (see p.129) • Check for congenital heart disease (see pp.118–119) • Undescended testes (see pp.160–161) • Vision (see pp.84–85 and pp.204–205) • Muscle tone • Reflexes (see p.15)
6–8 week check (by the doctor and health visitor)	• General physical examination • Height, weight and head circumference • Check for congenital dislocation of the hips • Check for congenital heart disease • Undescended testes • Whether your baby is smiling • Hearing and vision • Head control and muscle tone • Reflexes
7–9 month check (by the health visitor)	• Weight • General health • Hearing (see pp.86–87 and pp.202–203) • Developmental milestones for age (such as rolling, sitting, weight bearing, babbling, grasping and transferring objects) • Check for congenital dislocation of the hips • Eyes for squints and general vision
18–24 months (by the health visitor)	• Weight, gait and height • General health • Developmental milestones for age (such as scribbling, building with bricks and knowing body parts) • Emotion/behaviour • Speech and language • Vision and hearing
36–42 months (by the health visitor)	• Weight and height • General health • Developmental milestones for age (such as copying a cross, building with bricks and knowing colours) • Emotion/behaviour • Speech and language • Vision and hearing
48–66 months (by the doctor or school nurse before or when the child starts school)	• General physical examination (on a selective basis, depending on the child's health) • Weight and height • Vision and hearing • Development • Emotion/behaviour

SEE ALSO

Milestones	22–27
Speech and language problems	200–201
Learning difficulties	206–207

Breastfeeding

Health professionals strongly encourage breastfeeding, which provides important benefits for you and your baby. Breast milk contains the correct amounts of proteins, fats and carbohydrates that a baby needs for its development.

Breast milk also contains antibodies, which help to protect against gastroenteritis, coughs and colds, and urinary and ear infections. Constipation is uncommon in breastfed babies, and prolonged breastfeeding protects against eczema, food allergy and asthma. Breastfed children also have better

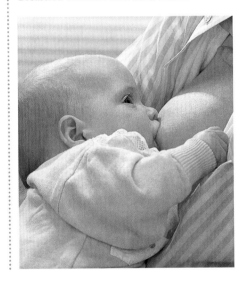

Breastfeeding your baby

Make sure that both you and your baby are comfortable when breastfeeding; correct positioning of your baby, or latching on, is important for successful feeding.

dental health, better eyesight and a higher IQ. In addition, breastfeeding helps you to regain your figure by using up the extra fat that is laid down in pregnancy.

Starting breastfeeding

Breastfeeding can take some time to get established and may not be easy at first, but with patience, and help from a health professional or breastfeeding organization, problems can usually be resolved. How your baby latches on to your breast is important. He is correctly positioned if:
- His mouth is wide open and his bottom lip is curled back and below the base of your nipple.
- He has a mouth full of breast – all of the nipple and most of the areola (the dark skin surrounding the nipple).
- His jaw muscles work rhythmically and the movement extends as far as his ears.

The main cause of sore nipples is an incorrect feeding position – check that your baby latches on properly. To help nipples heal, expose them to air or gently dry them with a hairdryer. Avoid soap, bubble bath, antiseptics and plastic-backed breast pads.

The more you feed, the more milk your breasts will make. Don't worry about timing feeds, but make sure you empty one breast completely before offering your baby the other. You will know he is getting enough milk if he is gaining weight and has six to eight wet nappies a day.

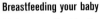

EXPRESSING MILK

You may wish to express milk if your baby is in the special care unit; if your breasts are engorged; if you are going out for several hours and someone else will feed your baby; or to store it if you are returning to work. Expressed breast milk can be stored in a sterile container in a refrigerator for 24 hours or a freezer for three months.

You can express milk by hand, or by using a hand pump, a battery pump or an electric pump. Not all women find expressing milk easy at first, but with practice it becomes easier. If you want to express by hand, ask another breastfeeding mother or a health professional to show you how if necessary. Before buying a pump, see if you can borrow or hire one first to make sure that it suits you.

Bottlefeeding

If you cannot breastfeed, you can bottlefeed your baby with an infant formula made from modified cow's milk. Ordinary cow's milk, goat's milk, evaporated or condensed milk are not suitable for babies under one year old.

Always follow the instructions when making a formula feed. Boil fresh tap water and, when it is cool, wash your hands, measure the water into a sterilized bottle and add the powder to the water. Before starting to feed, shake the bottle, then test the temperature of the milk by shaking a few drops on to your wrist – it should feel warm. If you plan to use the bottle later in the day, place the teat upside down in the bottle, cover the teat with a plastic disc, then cover it with a cap and place the bottle in the refrigerator. (Discard unused formula after 24 hours.)

Your baby needs about 150 g (2½ oz) of formula per kg (lb) of body weight a day. He may need feeding on demand or every two or three hours in the early weeks, and three to five times a day at six months of age. Never keep or reuse leftover milk.

TYPES OF MILK

Cow's milk-based formula is used for most bottlefed babies. In European Community countries, this must comply with a directive on its composition and contain certain levels of protein, carbohydrate, fats, vitamins and minerals. Formula milks (first milks) may be whey dominant and have protein similar to breast milk. Casein-dominant milks (second milks), based on whole cow's milk protein, tend to be used for hungry babies. The calorie content of both types of milk is the same.

Soya-based formula may be used if the baby cannot digest lactose or is allergic to cow's milk. It should be used only on the advice of a health professional. Specialized formulas are manufactured for babies with certain disorders or diseases.

Warm milk breeds bacteria, so bottles and teats must be kept scrupulously clean. Hand wash them before sterilizing, which can be done by boiling for 10 minutes or by steaming, using a microwave steam sterilizer or an electric steamer, or by immersion in a special chemical solution.

If your baby suffers from wind, check that the hole in the teat is neither too small nor too large to ensure that he is not sucking in extra air. It is common for a baby to posset, or bring up, a small amount of milk after feeding. If he is gaining weight, there is usually no cause for concern; it will improve when he is sitting and eating solids after six months.

Bottlefeeding your baby
Cuddle your baby on your lap, with his head and back supported by your arm. Tilt the bottle so that the teat is full of millk, not air.

Healthy family eating

Healthy eating is good for all the family, but a balanced diet is particularly important to meet your child's nutritional needs for energy and growth. Eating the wrong balance of foods can lead to problems in the long term.

The best way to provide a healthy, balanced diet for your child is to offer her a variety of foods each day from each of the four main food groups. Together, they contain all the essential nutrients – carbohydrates, protein, fat, vitamins and minerals.

The food groups

The first group includes bread, cereals, pasta, rice and potatoes. Beans and pulses can be eaten as part of this group, which is important for complex carbohydrates and also provides energy, fibre, protein, vitamins and minerals. Aim for one serving each mealtime for the under fives, more for older children.

Fruit and vegetables (including fresh, tinned and frozen), salads and fruit juice form the second group. They provide vitamins, particularly vitamin C, minerals and fibre. Aim for three to four servings daily for toddlers, five for older children. Fruit juice counts as only one serving, even if given more than once.

The third group incorporates meat, fish, eggs, pulses (peas, beans, canned baked beans and lentils), nuts (finely ground for the under fives; see box, opposite) and soya bean products. They supply protein, vitamins and minerals. Meat is a good source of iron. Fish includes fresh, frozen and canned fish and fish fingers. Aim for one serving daily from an animal source or two servings from a vegetable source.

Dairy products, such as milk, cheese, yogurt and butter – the fourth group – provide protein, fat, vitamins (especially A and D in whole-milk products) and minerals, especially calcium. Aim for about 350 ml (12 fl oz) of milk daily or two servings of dairy products for toddlers. Always give full-fat milk to children under the age of two.

The main food groups

A balanced diet should include foods from all the food groups: starchy foods – bread, cereals and rice – meat and fish; fruit and vegetables; and dairy products. A serving is a child-sized portion, about half or one-third of an adult's portion.

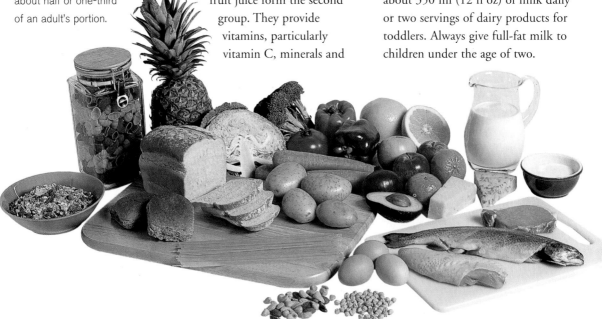

Weaning a baby

The process of ending a baby's total dependence on breast or formula milk and gradually introducing solid foods into her diet is known as weaning. It is important to start weaning your baby at the right time.

Health professionals generally recommend that weaning should start between four and six months. Starting to wean a baby before four months is not usually recommended because the digestive system is still immature and her kidneys may not be mature enough to deal with solid food. Introducing foods too early may also predispose her to allergies, and the muscle and nerve coordination needed for head control and to enable her to swallow food may not be fully developed.

Starting to wean a baby after six months is not recommended because after this age she needs more iron and other nutrients than milk can provide. If you leave it too long, she will find it more difficult to learn to chew and may not accept new tastes and textures so readily.

Starting weaning

Take things slowly. Choose a time when your baby is not too tired and you are not feeling rushed such as during lunch. Give her some milk from the breast or bottle before offering her a spoon or two of food. Suitable first foods include baby rice; puréed fruit, such as banana, peeled and cooked pear, apple and apricots (don't add sugar); and puréed vegetables such as potatoes, parsnips and carrots (boiled without salt).

Once your baby is used to a spoon, slowly increase the amount of food and add others, such as soft cooked meats and pulses, more vegetables and fruit and full-fat yogurt. Work up to giving food two or three times daily. Also give at least 560 ml (1 pint) of breast or formula milk up to the age of 12 months.

From six to nine months, mash or mince foods to encourage your baby to chew, and introduce a wider range – for example, meat, well-cooked egg, porridge, baked beans and fish. Introduce finger foods, such as toast, pasta and cubes of fruit, vegetables and hard cheese.

By 9 to 12 months, your baby should be on three meals a day, with snacks in between. Most meals can be the same as those of the rest of the family – her food needs only to be cut into small pieces.

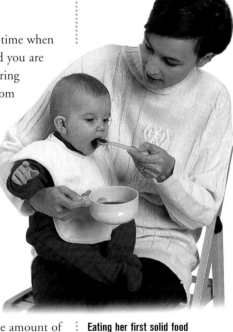

Eating her first solid food
Your main aim when weaning your child is to introduce new tastes and to teach her to eat from a spoon. If she doesn't take food at first, don't insist but try again a week later.

FOODS TO AVOID

For the first six months:
- Gluten (look for "gluten free" on baby food labels)
- Citrus fruit
- Eggs
- Nuts (if there is a family history of allergies, avoid peanuts until the age of five)

For the first 12 months:
- Liver pâté and unpasteurized soft cheeses
- Honey (on rare occasions, this may cause a potentially serious illness called infant botulism).

Feeding a toddler

Toddlers have high daily requirements for energy (calories) and other nutrients, but they cannot eat large amounts of food at a sitting, and their eating habits may be poor. They need three small meals a day, with snacks in between.

Family eating

Toddlers can be fussy when it comes to eating, and they may refuse to eat many foods. Rather than pressuring your child to eat, sit her with the rest of the family at the dinner table, where she may join in when she sees others enjoying their meal.

Toddlers need to obtain their calories and nutrients from a balanced diet, but it should differ from a diet for adults. They need fat because it is a concentrated source of energy and vitamins, and it provides essential fatty acids. The best sources are full-fat milk, cheese and other dairy foods, meat and eggs – these foods contain fats in an easily digested, concentrated form, and they provide other nutrients such as calcium and iron.

Don't give your toddler too many high-fibre foods. These may fill him up, so that he does not want other more nutritious foods. A high-fibre diet may also lead to diarrhoea and can interfere with absorption of minerals such as iron.

You can give vitamin A, C and D drops to children under five, unless they are eating a good diet. Try to give some iron-containing foods every day and increase iron absorption by giving food or fruit juice containing vitamin C at every meal.

Getting your toddler to eat

Children are faddy eaters but no one food is essential to health. If you offer a variety of foods from the four food groups, even over the course of several days, he is likely to be getting a balanced diet.

If your child won't eat fruit, try adding cream, full-fat yogurt, custard or dairy ice cream to it. Add butter to vegetables and mashed or jacket potatoes. Calcium is vital for healthy bones and teeth. If he won't drink milk, add it to cereals or give him other dairy products instead.

Healthy snacks

Most children need snacks between meals. Healthy snacks include:
- Fresh fruit (peeled and cut into slices for babies or toddlers); raw vegetables such as carrots, peppers, cucumber or celery; small chunks of cheese and pineapple; celery filled with cream cheese
- Fruitcake; carrot cake; rice cakes with or without a spread; buttered scone or bun; breadsticks; malt or fruit bread
- Unsweetened yogurt; unsweetened breakfast cereals, with or without milk
- Drink of whole milk or well-diluted unsweetened pure fruit juice.

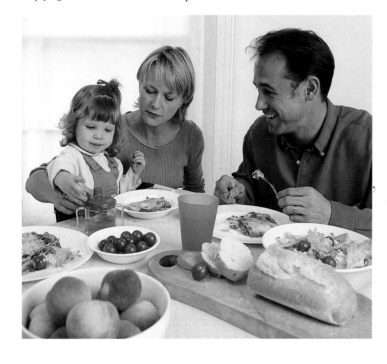

Feeding a schoolchild

Like the preschool child, schoolchildren who are still growing need a well-balanced diet to supply their energy and other nutrients. Many of the dietary guidelines and healthy snacks suggested for toddlers also apply to them.

As your child gets older, it can be more difficult to keep a watch on what he eats. Frequent snacking or grazing on sugary foods and drinks is often preferred to a proper meal. But as with toddlers, encourage him to eat healthy snacks and drinks, and don't let him fill up on cakes, crisps and biscuits.

Studies have also found that eating breakfast, especially one of fortified cereal, is important for schoolchildren, so make sure that he eats a proper meal in the morning before he goes off to school.

A packed lunch may be one of your child's three main meals if he doesn't take school meals, so it needs to provide plenty of nutrients. It should contain food from at least three of the four main food groups, which is also interesting, varied and enjoyable, so that he will eat it.

LUNCH BOX SUGGESTIONS

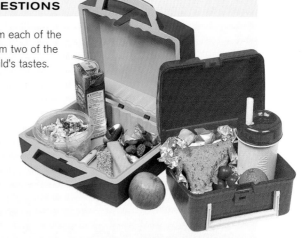

- Sandwiches, rolls or pitta bread with two types of filling, one from each of the two columns below, provide a contrast and also contain food from two of the food groups. You can mix and match them, according to your child's tastes.

cream cheese	dates or crushed pineapple
grated cheese	fruit chutney
peanut butter	sliced banana
cold chicken	avocado
tuna	sweetcorn and mayonnaise
salmon	cucumber
cold roast pork	apple
bacon	lettuce and tomato
egg	watercress
ham	salad
fish pâté	tomato

- Alternatives to sandwiches: containers can be filled with pasta, potato or rice, mixed with natural yogurt, fromage frais or mayonnaise. Add food such as cold chicken chunks; chopped apples or celery; tuna; chopped fresh tomatoes and kidney beans; chunks of cheese, pineapple and salad. Cold pizza with various mixed toppings, such as cheese, tomatoes, ham, pineapple, mushrooms, pepperoni or tuna.

- Dairy foods: carton of yogurt or fromage frais; tub of cheese cubes (with grapes or pineapple chunks); pot of cottage cheese; cheese dip with vegetable sticks or a bread stick.

- Fruits and vegetables: add loose or put into a tub cherry tomatoes, grapes or raw vegetables, such as sticks of celery, carrot, pepper and cucumber (with a dip if you wish); tub of fruit salad; apple, banana, peach, satsuma or other piece of fruit.

- Suitable drinks: milk or yogurt drink; pure unsweetened fruit juice; water.

- Treats: Yogurt- or chocolate-coated nuts and raisins; crisps or other savoury snacks; muesli bar.

Note: items with mayonnaise and some dairy foods should only be kept in insulated lunch boxes or with gel-type ice packs to keep food and drinks cool.

Teeth and tooth care

The number of under-fives with no tooth decay has risen, but children who do have problems have more serious decay and need more fillings. Looking after your child's teeth will pay dividends in preventing tooth decay.

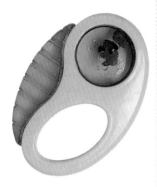

Teething ring
You can help reduce the pain of teething by giving your child a gel-type teething ring to chew on. For the best effect, first cool it in the refrigerator.

Baby's first teeth
The first teeth are the two lower incisors (1) – the middle teeth in the lower gum – followed by the two upper incisors (2), then the rest of the incisors (3). These are followed by the first molars (4), then the canines (5). The second bottom molars (6) come through at 20 months, followed by the top molars (7).

Most babies start to cut their first tooth around the age of six months, although the teeth start to develop under the gums between six and eight weeks after conception. Some babies are born with one or more teeth. Most children have three or four by their first birthday (although it is not unusual to have none at all at this stage) and all 20 first, or milk, teeth by the age of three.

Between the ages of six and eight, the first teeth start to fall out, a process that is usually complete by the age of 11 or 12. Your child will not, however, have his full complement of 32 permanent teeth until his late teens.

As the teeth break through, your baby may experience some discomfort. Signs that your baby may be teething are if she is irritable or fretful; dribbles a great deal;

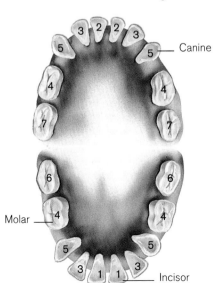

Canine

Molar

Incisor

gnaws at hard objects or chews her fingers; or has flushed cheeks. Illness such as diarrhoea, vomiting, fever and signs of earache are not due to teething.

Relieving discomfort

If your baby is uncomfortable while she is teething, give her plenty of extra cuddles and try these measures.
- A sugar-free teething gel may help relieve red and sore gums.
- Gently rub the gums with your finger or a small chip of ice.
- Give your baby something hard to chew on, such as a crust of bread or a carrot, or offer a chilled teething ring.
- A dose of paracetamol may help. Use it sparingly and follow the instructions regarding dosage. (Never give a child under the age of 12 aspirin; see p.63.)
- Try a teething remedy such as chamomile teething drops.
- Give your baby plenty of cool drinks.
- Relieve a teething rash on the cheeks, or one under the chin that has been caused by dribbling, by applying petroleum jelly.

Preventing tooth decay

Your child's first teeth are just as important as her permanent teeth. Decay of the first teeth is painful and requires dental work – either filling or removal. If the first teeth are lost too soon, your child's second teeth may grow crooked or they may be overcrowded and result in your child needing braces or extractions later on. To help avoid tooth decay in your baby, discourage her from drinking milk from a bottle after the age of one, never let her drink juice from a bottle and don't use dummies filled with fluid.

Diet and the teeth

A balanced diet is vital to provide your child with the nutrients that she needs for the growth and development of healthy teeth and gums. Protein, vitamins and the minerals calcium, phosphorus and fluoride are essential for well-formed, decay-resistant teeth and gums.

The main cause of tooth decay is frequent intake of refined sugars. Look for "hidden" sugars such as sucrose, glucose, dextrose, lactose, fructose (fruit sugars, which are particularly concentrated in dried fruit such as raisins), honey, caramel or syrups in various foods, and limit your child's exposure to them. Sugar is most damaging when consumed frequently throughout the day. It is less damaging when eaten as part of a meal, because fats have a buffering effect and saliva helps to wash away sugar from the tooth surface, as well as to remineralize tooth enamel.

Limit your child's intake of sugary snacks and drinks and encourage her to eat healthy snacks. Sticky sweets, such as nougat, toffee and caramel, and dried fruits are particularly likely to adhere to the tooth surface. Boiled sweets, chewing gum containing sugar, mints and lollies expose the tooth surfaces to sugar over a longer period of time. If your child consumes sugary foods and drinks between meals, some dentists advise brushing the teeth afterward. Or allow your child to chew sugar-free gum to stimulate the flow of saliva.

To avoid erosion, encourage children to:
● Drink plain water, milk or diluted fruit juice rather than squash and carbonated drinks, which contain citric, phosphoric or malic acids.
● Only drink beverages from a straw that is placed behind the top front teeth.
● Do not sip sugary beverages slowly or swish acid drinks around in the mouth.

Going to the dentist

From the age of three your child should visit the dentist regularly every six months, but some dentists like to check a child's teeth at two years old. At first, you can take your child with you when you go for a check up so she gets used to the dentist and surgery. At her first visit, the dentist will check for any signs of decay or other problems and give you advice on oral health. Regular dental check ups will ensure that your child's teeth remain healthy and that any signs of decay or other dental problems are detected early.

LOOKING AFTER YOUR BABY'S TEETH

Use a fluoride toothpaste formulated for children and a soft baby toothbrush when your child's teeth first appear. From about the age of three your child may want to brush his teeth himself, but you should continue to do so too until he is at least school age.

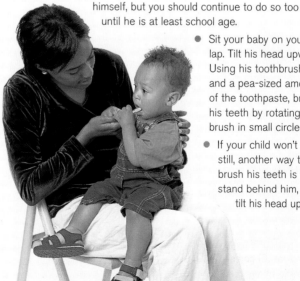

● Sit your baby on your lap. Tilt his head upward. Using his toothbrush and a pea-sized amount of the toothpaste, brush his teeth by rotating the brush in small circles.

● If your child won't sit still, another way to brush his teeth is to stand behind him, and tilt his head upward.

Feet and foot care

Most babies are born with normal feet, but many children go on to develop foot problems as adults. However, with proper care and attention, there is no reason why your child should not enter adulthood with perfect feet.

There are 26 small bones in the feet which are held together by ligaments, tendons and muscles. These are all present at birth, but are mainly composed of soft tissue and cartilage. As the feet grow, the cartilage ossifies and becomes bone, but the bones of a child's feet are not fully formed until he is 18 or 19 years old.

Consequently, children's feet are soft and pliable, and the toes can easily be deformed if they are bent or moulded into the wrong shape – for example, by wearing poorly fitting shoes and socks. As your baby grows, check that socks and the feet of sleepsuits and tights are not too tight and don't restrict the feet. If necessary, cut the toe area off the sleepsuits to allow his feet to move freely.

Keeping feet healthy
Allow your child to walk around barefoot at home to help develop his walking muscles.

Don't tuck your baby's bedclothes in too tightly – he needs room to exercise his feet by kicking and wriggling.

A baby doesn't need shoes. In fact, shoes are not necessary until your child is ready to walk outdoors, and even then you can let him walk outdoors barefoot whenever it is safe to do so – such as on grass in your back garden, where you know there won't be broken glass and it won't have been fouled by an animal.

Buying shoes

It is important that shoes fit properly. Even when buying summer shoes such as sandals, your child's feet should be measured. When you buy shoes make sure that there is room for growth, but don't buy shoes half a size bigger for your child to grow into. Check the shoe while your child is standing and get him to walk across the room to test for comfort. Then get him to stand on tiptoe. If the heel slips off, a smaller size is needed.

Children's feet grow quickly, especially during the second and third years, but because there is so little bone in a child's foot he may not complain about shoes that are too small hurting him. After

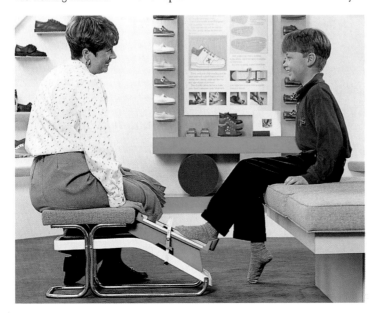

Getting a proper fit
Buy shoes from a shop that specializes in a children's fitting service. Make sure both feet are measured – one foot may be a different size or width to the other.

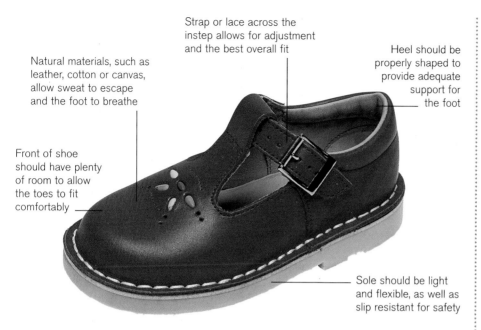

Strap or lace across the instep allows for adjustment and the best overall fit

Natural materials, such as leather, cotton or canvas, allow sweat to escape and the foot to breathe

Heel should be properly shaped to provide adequate support for the foot

Front of shoe should have plenty of room to allow the toes to fit comfortably

Sole should be light and flexible, as well as slip resistant for safety

SEE ALSO
Bones, muscles
and joints   **120–121**
Flat feet   **130**
Talipes   **131**

First shoes
When buying a child's shoes make sure they fit properly along the length, width and girth of the foot. There should be one finger's width between the big toe and the front of the shoe.

buying shoes for your child, check them again in eight weeks to make sure they still fit. If he needs new ones, have his feet measured again. Children should never wear secondhand shoes or those passed down from one child to another. Don't keep a pair of expensive shoes "for best" for long; your child may grow out of them before he has a chance to wear them.

As your child grows older and more fashion conscious, he will probably demand the latest trendy shoes. Shoes such as trainers and boots are not bad for the feet if they are made of natural materials and fit properly, but don't allow your child to wear sloppy casual shoes all day. If your child wants to wear stylish shoes with sharply pointed toes or high heels, they should be reserved for special occasions – not everyday wear.

Care of the feet
Once your child starts walking, you may need to wash his feet more often. Warm soapy water is all that is needed, but take particular care to dry your child's feet properly, especially between the toes to

help avoid problems such as athlete's foot (see p.108). As your child gets older and baths himself, remind him to dry his feet properly. When you wash your child's feet, inspect them for problems such as warts (see p.107), rashes, blisters (see p.105), changes in colour or any cuts.

Insist that your child wear clean socks daily; those containing natural fibres such as cotton or wool are best. Make sure, too, that they are the correct size. Socks that are too big can bunch and cause pressure on your child's foot. If they are too small, they will constrict the foot and bend the toes.

GROWTH AND MEASUREMENT GUIDE

- On average, a child's feet will grow two full shoe sizes every year between one and four years of age.
- The average growth rate is one full shoe size a year between 5 and 10 years of age.
- Girls' feet stop growing between the ages of 10 and 14 years; boys feet, between 14 and 18 years.
- As a general guide, children's feet should be measured at: 6 to 8 week intervals for children under four years of age and 10 to 12 week intervals for children over four years old.

Hair care

Some babies are born with a full head of hair, others are bald or have just a few tufts. Almost all new babies lose some or all of their hair by the fourth month, when the mature hair comes in, so your baby may briefly be bald.

The hair on a newborn is different in colour and texture from the hair that grows later on. The rate of hair growth is about 1 cm (½ in) a month, but at 12 months some children are still bald, while others have a mop of hair. There may be a bald patch at the back of the head where the baby sleeps on it – it will disappear as the baby gets older.

Washing a child's hair

Caring for your baby's hair is simple. It does not need washing every day; when it does, it can be washed when you bath her (see pp.16–17). At other times, tidy the hair by wiping it with a damp cloth and brushing it with a soft baby brush.

As your child grows, washing her hair can become more difficult. Many children hate getting water on their face or are frightened of shampoo stinging their eyes; you should avoid adult shampoos and use a mild or non-sting shampoo. If your daughter has long hair, you can try using a spray-on conditioner that won't need rinsing out. If you still have difficulty getting your child to cooperate, when she is in the bath ask her to lie back and wet her hair in the water. Quickly shampoo it when she sits up, then use a jug of water or spray attachment to rinse her hair, with her head tilted backward.

Another option is to try to turn hair washing into a game. Let your child pour water over her head with a container or the shower spray and use lots of mild bubble bath in the water. Encourage your child to rub this over her head and make her laugh by showing her the effect in a mirror. Then let her pour water over her head and check in the mirror that all the bubbles have gone.

If your child really refuses to have her hair washed without a struggle, keep it short and sponge it with a damp cloth regularly, until she is willing to have it washed. Or if she is old enough, she may enjoy going to the hairdresser's to have it washed and trimmed.

Brushing a child's hair

To keep long hair free from tangles, you will have to brush it regularly; however, if the hair is wet, you should always use a wide-tooth comb. If you braid your daughter's hair or put it in bunches, be careful not to pull her hair back too tightly. This could make the hair fall out or cause thinning or permanent bald patches. You should also avoid using rubber bands – hair can easily become tangled and knotted in them.

It is common for young babies to have cradle cap, and as children get older, for them to catch head lice. You should remember that these conditions are not related to poor hygiene and are no reflection on your care of your child's hair.

Protective shield

If your child makes a fuss when it comes to washing her hair, it may be because she fears soap getting into her eyes – try using a hair shield to protect them.

Nail care

A newborn's nails are often much longer than new parents expect. To prevent the baby from scratching herself, the nails need to be trimmed to keep them short and smooth – or they can be covered with mittens.

SEE ALSO
Bathing your baby and
helping him to sleep   16–17
Worms   97
Your child's skin   100–101

A good time to trim a baby's nails is just after a bath, when they will be soft; however, you may find it easier to trim them when she is asleep. In the early weeks, her fingernails may need trimming as often as twice a week. As your child gets older, check her fingernails at regular intervals and cut them before they become too long. Keeping nails short and clean is especially important when your child starts nursery or school, because long nails increase the chances of her catching threadworms.

Toenails tend to grow more slowly than fingernails, so you may only need to trim them once or twice a month. They are usually soft and pliable in a young baby, but will become harder as she grows up.

NAIL BITING

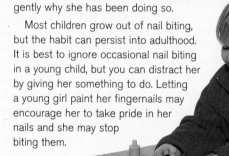

About one-third of all children pick up the habit of biting their nails. A child may bite her nails when she is concentrating on something else, such as television, and may not realize she is doing it. On its own, nail biting does not indicate any severe emotional problems, but it is a way of relieving tension. If you find that your child has bitten her nails, ask her gently why she has been doing so.

Most children grow out of nail biting, but the habit can persist into adulthood. It is best to ignore occasional nail biting in a young child, but you can distract her by giving her something to do. Letting a young girl paint her fingernails may encourage her to take pride in her nails and she may stop biting them.

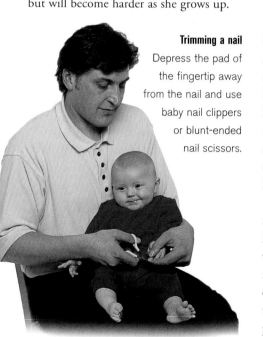

Trimming a nail
Depress the pad of the fingertip away from the nail and use baby nail clippers or blunt-ended nail scissors.

Ingrown nails

A toenail can become ingrown when the edge of the nail cuts into the skin, leaving it red and hard and sometimes infected. Ingrown nails are more common in teenagers than in young children. If you are concerned that your child may have an ingrown nail, you should talk to your health professional.

To avoid creating an ingrown nail, make sure that you or your child don't leave a spike at the edge of the nail when cutting it. Chiropodists now recommend that toenails are cut in a curved line, following the contour of the toe – not straight across as was previously recommended.

Safety in the home

Most accidents involving young children occur in the home and the most common ones are falls, cuts and bruises. From the time your child is born, you will need to think and behave differently in your own home.

Natural curiosity

Young children like to explore and experiment, so it is important that all cleaning products are kept either in a cupboard with a lock or in one that is high up, out of their reach.

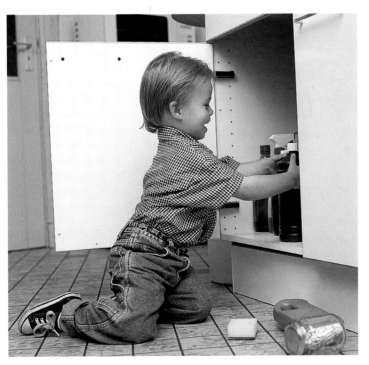

Even naturally cautious parents will have to make adjustments in their home to make it safe for a young child. Start by reviewing your house as a whole. If you have not already installed smoke alarms, do so immediately. Check that the structure of your house is safe: make sure windows are secure in their frames and locked, and cover glass doors with a safety film so that if the glass does break, it won't shatter everywhere.

While you are reviewing your home in this light, remember not to underestimate what a young child can achieve in terms of exploration, even before he can walk or stand unaided. Store glass and other fragile ornaments out of reach. Fit safety covers into any unused electrical sockets. To prevent your child from skidding on sliding rugs, fit anti-slip runners to them or tape them down. Invest in stairguards for both the top and bottom of any stairs, and make sure stair carpets are well attached for when your child is old enough to use the stairs. Low cost safety equipment loans may be available; ask for details from your health care visitor.

Making your kitchen safe

The kitchen is the key area for accidents in the home, but they can be avoided by following safety procedures at all times. Children learn by example from an early age and will not respond to instructions or warnings if they see you taking risks.

Before your child can crawl, inspect the room for any potential hazards. Store cleaning products in lockable or out-of-reach cupboards and keep sharp knives out of reach. Secure doors on large appliances and keep flexes out of reach. If you have toddlers, bins need a childproof catch. Don't use a tablecloth, which your child can pull on top of himself, along with everything on the cloth.

Never leave a child alone in the kitchen when the oven is on. If you buy a new oven, choose one with a stay-cool door. Place saucepans on the back hobs when you can; when using the front hobs, turn handles in so they can't be grabbed. Never leave hot drinks within reach of a child, including in other rooms. Ensure the area where you prepare hot drinks is free from clutter so you are less likely to spill fluids.

At hectic times, place a baby or toddler in a playpen and discourage an older child from hovering next to you and the cooker. Provide a corner of the kitchen where he can safely sit and talk to you, or insist that he waits until you have finished cooking. Never allow a toddler to use tricycles or trolleys in the kitchen.

If your child is keen to learn how to make tea or coffee, it is for you to judge his readiness. Do not go by his age or make comparisons with what he says his peers are doing. Each child develops at an individual rate. Without frightening him or taking away his desire to experience everything, approach cooking tasks, such as boiling a kettle of water, turning on the cooker or using the microwave oven, with a sensible amount of caution. Do not assume that because you have shown your child how to do something once, he will remember it the next time. Go through the routine a few times, and keep an eye on what he is doing until you are sure he understands the safety issues.

Around the house

Look around your living room for items that can be pulled down or knocked over, including lightweight furniture, and fit protectors on sharp furniture corners. Hide or tape down any wires, and move small objects out of reach. Tie curtain, blind or shade cords out of reach to avoid strangulation. Invest in a fire screen that fits to the wall, and move furniture that can be climbed upon away from windows. Remove any poisonous house plants.

If you use a car seat or baby bouncer in the house, always place it on the floor, never on a raised surface. Never leave a baby on beds or sofas, from which he

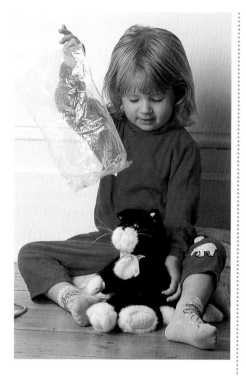

might fall to the floor. If your baby can move about, keep duvets, pillows and cushions out of reach to avoid smothering and overheating. Keep wardrobe doors shut and locked to prevent adventurous toddlers from entering them.

Train pets to stay out of bedrooms to avoid the risk of the animal sleeping on top of the child and smothering him. Treat animals for flea and worm infestation on a regular basis, but still teach children not to play with feeding bowls or bedding.

SEE ALSO
Sudden infant death syndrome   18–19
Burns   216
Poisoning   217

Plastic alert
Young children can suffocate by playing with plastic bags, which they sometimes like to put over their heads. Always remove and keep all plastic bags out of your child's reach.

BATHROOM SAFETY

You should take the following precautions in the bathroom:
- Never leave a baby or toddler alone in the bath; he can drown in as little as 8 cm (3 in) of water.
- Keep medicines, nail polish remover and other potential poisons locked in a cupboard, out of reach of your child. Make sure you know what to do if your child swallows a dangerous substance.
- Check the thermostat on your water heater. Water that is hotter than 48°C (118°F) can scald a baby.
- Make sure the lock on the door can be unlocked from outside.

Safety in the garden

The garden can become your child's own little kingdom, where she can explore to her heart's content and create exciting adventures, but first you need to ensure that your garden is hazard-free.

Make security a priority. There should be no gaps in hedges through which small children can escape and fences should be too high to climb – the recommended height is 1,200 mm (4 ft). Keep all gates locked, especially if near a road. Dispose of all rubbish in a place inaccessible to the child, so that she can't cut herself on broken glass or sharp cans. Make it a firm rule to keep the garden tidy and put everything away after use.

You should always store weedkillers, insecticides and other chemicals in their original containers and lock them away well out of your child's reach. You should never store them in other containers, such as washing-up liquid bottles, so that there can be no mistake about what's in them. Garden chemicals are toxic and a child can be poisoned, even by a tiny amount. The main risk to a child is usually if she accidentally swallows a chemical; however, some chemicals can be harmful if only inhaled. If you have to use a weedkiller or a similar chemical in the garden, always do so when your children are safely in the house.

Garden tools should always be locked away when not in use; switch off and put away any electrical equipment as soon as it is no longer needed. You should never leave an upright ladder unattended – most young children will find the urge to climb it irresistible.

Don't use stakes or canes for your plants anywhere near where your children play, and be careful of where you position shrubs that will need pruning. A sharp, pruned branch can puncture the skin of a child who falls on it. Of course, position any plants with sharp thorns out of reach of children too.

The garden is often the venue for family parties, and barbecues are always popular. It's important to keep small children away from the barbecue area while you are cooking, and don't leave it unattended until it has cooled down. The same applies to a bonfire, which should be put out and not left to burn down.

DANGEROUS PLANTS

A very young child often puts things straight into her mouth, while an older child may pull up plants and play with them. Some plants can be harmful to your child if they are eaten or handled. If you have any of the following plants, you should remove them from your garden:

- Autumn crocus (*Colchicum autumnale*)
- Flannel bush (*Fremontodendron*)
- Foxglove (*Digitalis purpurea*)
- Ivy (*Hedera*)
- Laburnum (*Laburnum*)
- Leyland cypress (*Cupressocyparis leylandii*)
- Lily of the valley (*Convallaria*)
- Lupins (*Lupinus*)
- Mezereon (*Daphne mezereum*)
- Monkshood (*Aconitum*)
- Pokeweed (*Phytolacca*)
- Rue (*Ruta*)
- Spurge (*Euphorbia*)
- Yew (*Taxus baccata*)

This is not an exhaustive list, so discourage your child from putting things in her mouth. When choosing new garden plants and shrubs don't hesitate to ask the advice of the staff at the garden centre.

IS YOUR GARDEN SAFE?

Before letting your child play in the garden, inspect it carefully for any potential hazards.

- Fence off or cover any pools and ponds with mesh.
- Make sure garden gates and fences are secure.
- Remove any poisonous plants.
- Always keep garden tools and chemicals locked up.
- Ensure that large play equipment, such as a climbing frame or swing, is firmly secured.
- Remove any garden and building rubbish, and keep rubbish bins securely covered.

Make sure you keep the matches well out of reach. As an extra precaution keep a bucket of sand nearby to extinguish any unexpected flares.

Garden features

Water is fascinating to small children, but it is also dangerous. Your toddler could drown in only 8 cm (3 in) of water, so supervise her whenever she is near a pond or water butt or playing in a paddling pool. You should cover ponds, water butts and other containers that can collect rainwater, but you still need to be vigilant because children have been known to drown in covered ponds. Always empty the paddling pool as soon as your child has finished playing in it. You'll need to be even more cautious when visiting other homes.

A child-friendly garden is likely to have some permanent play equipment – a swing, slide or climbing frame. Ensure that you buy equipment of an appropriate height for your child's size and age, and be prepared to replace it with more challenging equipment as she grows. You can limit the risk of bumps, bruises and serious head injuries caused by falls by providing a soft, safe play surface under the play equipment. Grass is the normal choice in most family gardens but sand, bark or rubber tiles are even better.

All play structures must be fixed firmly into the ground and require regular inspection for wear and tear. When siting swings and climbing frames, make sure they are well away from trees, bushes and glass structures such as greenhouses.

Older children may want a tree house. As long as it is a firm structure, situated at a reasonable height and the access is made as secure as possible, it should not pose a problem. Ensure your child understands safety issues, and don't allow too many children in the tree house at one time.

A favourite piece of garden play equipment among toddlers is the sandpit. Keep a sandpit in the garden covered when not in use so that neighbourhood cats do not use it as a litter tray.

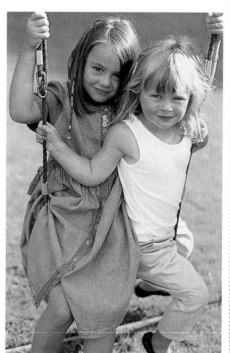

SEE ALSO
Bleeding   216
Poisoning   217
Broken bones   218–219
Head injuries   219

Swing safety
Most children enjoy playing on a swing. A toddler will require adult supervision, but once you are confident that your child knows to hold on, you can allow her to swing by herself.

Street safety

A child's ability to function safely in the streets and to feel confident in any situations that may arise will often grow out of your own attitude and behaviour when you first take him outdoors as a baby.

Padded protection

Whether your child prefers rollerblades or a skateboard, she should always wear a helmet and knee and elbow pads. It is also a good idea for her to wear wrist guards.

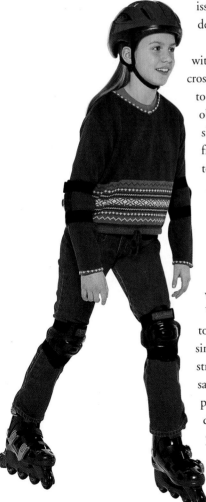

You should find time to go out with your child without the car. Many children are driven to nursery or school, delivered to friends' houses in the car and brought back home the same way. Most of these journeys are under 3 km (1½ miles) and have the negative effects of reducing your child's independence and increasing air pollution – an important issue since more children are developing asthma (see pp.76–77).

When you undertake journeys with a pushchair, always use pedestrian crossings and, even if you were prone to take risks before you were a parent, obey road safety rules. You will be slower with a pushchair and, apart from the risk to your child, he needs to learn how to cross a street safely. As your child gets older, talk him through the procedure each time you follow it. Tell him to find a safe place to cross the road; stop, look in both directions and listen for cars; let traffic pass; and only when the road is clear walk across. You may find walking with a toddler tedious at times, especially since most toddlers are curious. Wrist straps or a harness and reins are useful safety aids. Remember to adapt your pace to your child's so he is not discouraged, and allow extra time for your outings so that you do not feel frustrated. Always ensure your child walks on the inside of the

kerb and holds your hand if you are not using a strap or reins. It's easy to become distracted if you're with more than one child; however, it is more important to pay attention to safety than to the children's conversation.

Walking alone

When your child gets older you should gently guide him toward independence. Walking on his own to school is often the first trip a child asks to make when he becomes aware that some of his peers are doing so. You should accompany your child at first, but let him decide where to cross the roads and which way to go.

Only when you are satisfied that he has developed road safety awareness should you allow him to go alone – there is a much greater risk from road accidents than from abduction. If your child intends to walk with friends, you need to be sure that he won't become so involved in conversation that he'll forget to follow road safety. Fluorescent strips for clothing are useful if he is walking home on dark winter afternoons, especially if you live in a rural setting.

Whether or not your child walks to school, he should become familiar with his surroundings and be able to visit shops, friends or neighbours alone. As with any journey, accompany him at first to increase awareness of potential danger such as blind spots in the road or lonely alleyways that should be avoided. Keep

this issue in an undramatic way. If an approach is made by someone in a car, tell your child to step back from the vehicle so that he cannot be grabbed and to insist loudly that he cannot help the driver before running in the opposite direction from the one that the car is pointing in.

Travelling on wheels

Your child will inevitably use the streets with a bicycle, rollerblades or skateboard. With cycling, impress upon him that he is in charge of a vehicle, not a toy. Using the roads requires training. Ask his school or the local police about cycling proficiency courses. Become acquainted with bicycle parts and how to keep them in safe working order. Faulty brakes, lights and chains are hazards. Of course, it is pointless having this knowledge if your child refuses to wear a safety helmet and reflective flashes on clothes – this is something you must be firm about.

With rollerblading or skateboarding, ensure that your child wears pads and a helmet at all times and that he goes only where it is safe to do so.

SEE ALSO

Safety in the home	44–45
Safety in the garden	46–47
Promoting your child's development: under 5	50–51

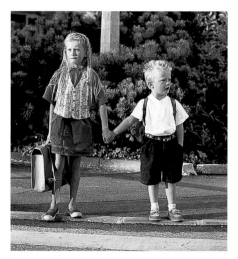

Crossing the road

Teach your children to use pedestrian crossings, and make sure they look in both directions before they step off the kerb.

your advice calm and to the point so that your child is not deterred.

When your child is old enough to go further afield, equip him with a telephone card and teach him to use public pay phones, or give him a mobile phone. Prepare your child for an emergency by instructing him to shout loudly and call "help" to passers-by if necessary. Discuss

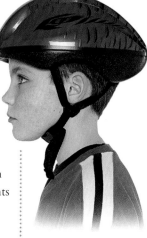

Helmet safety

Make sure the helmet fits snugly and sits level on the head – not tilted to the front or back. The chin strap should always be tightly secured.

CAR SAFETY

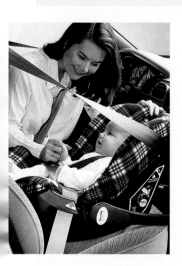

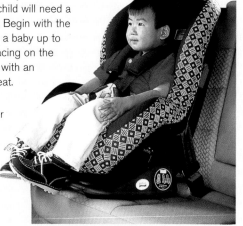

When travelling in a car, a child must always be in a suitable restraint for his age and weight. Your child will need a different type of restraint as he grows. Begin with the baby carrier (left), which is suitable for a baby up to nine months old. You can use it rear facing on the front passenger seat in cars not fitted with an airbag; otherwise use it on the back seat.

Use a car seat (right) for a child up to 4 years old, then switch to a booster seat for children under 11 years old. Anchor the seat or booster on the back seat with a seat belt.

Never buy a secondhand restraint – it may have been previously damaged and may no longer function safely.

Promoting your child's development: under 5

As a parent, you are uniquely qualified to set your child on the road to academic success. There are practical ways that you can help, starting in the first weeks of life.

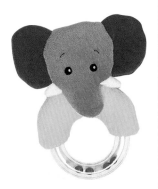

Animal-shaped rattle
An old favourite, the rattle is still one of the most effective ways of giving the child auditory and visual stimulation.

In the first five years of a child's life, all learning will take place through play, so one of the most important things you can do is to encourage your child to play. Research shows that children who are given a wide range of playthings – the "tools" for learning – are better prepared to reach higher levels of intellectual development, regardless of their sex, race and social class.

You should ensure that all your child's toys, games and books are appropriate for her age and capabilities. Items that are too advanced will only cause frustration, while anything that is not challenging enough will simply be seen as boring and be ignored by the child.

Birth to one year
In the first few weeks of life, a baby will enjoy focusing on objects that move or are patterned. Nursery mobiles should be hung about 20 cm (8 in) away from the baby in the first couple of months because anything further away will appear blurred to her. She will also be interested in a string of brightly coloured objects strung across her cot or pram, and when she is

Building blocks
By the time a toddler reaches 18 months, she can usually manage to build a tower using at least three blocks.

between three and four months old she will reach out and try to grasp them. An activity centre that can be attached to the side of the cot is a good choice. It should be brightly coloured and include a number of activities – different textures for tactile experiences, shiny mirrors in which she can see herself and items to turn and press that produce interesting sounds. Once your baby is sitting up unaided, she will enjoy building blocks and large beakers for stacking.

One to two years
Give her simple shape sorters and construction toys to help develop her hand–eye coordination and manipulative skills. You can make up a "treasure basket" that includes a variety of small, safe household items – for example, cotton reels, saucepan lids and pieces of fabric with a strong tactile quality such as velvet

Interactive playmat
An activity quilt is ideal for babies between 3 and 18 months old. Choose one that makes noises and has bright colours, mirrors and removable shapes.

or satin. Vary the contents frequently so that your baby doesn't become bored. You can encourage first words with a toy telephone, and finger puppets are fun for simulating conversation.

Two to three years

Her manipulative skills are developing rapidly, and she should now be able to complete simple jigsaws. She will like to imitate grown-up behaviour, so this is the time when a toy tea set, pretend cooking utensils, a miniature carpet sweeper or garden tools and a wheelbarrow really come into their own. Dolls of all types and sizes offer lots of play potential for both girls and boys. She should be provided with plenty of thick crayons and finger paints for her first works of art.

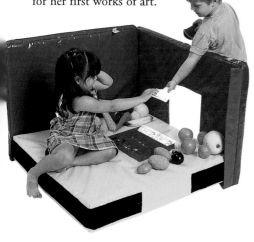

Three to four years

At this age role play becomes very imaginative and dressing up clothes are essential. Provide a selection of hats, old curtains (which make great cloaks), floaty scarves and extra props such as discarded spectacles with the lenses removed. Buy her a playhouse that easily converts into a shop, bank or even a hairdresser's. Your child will now begin to enjoy simple board games that encourage basic counting and observational skills.

Four to five years

She is able to recognize and probably write her own name, and the more able child will know several words or even read simple texts. In order to encourage preliteracy skills, make sure your child has a constant supply of pens, pencils, crayons, paintbrushes and paint. You will find that she does lots of pretend writing, even if none of it yet includes identifiable letters. Give her old diaries or cheque stubs to play with, and make use of the junk mail that comes through the letterbox by cutting out coupons and forms for her to "fill in".

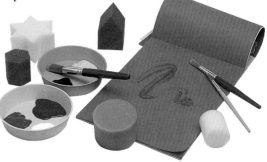

Playing shop

Your children can use a simple "room" as a shop or office for creative role playing. A few extra props, such as some vegetables and fruit, can make their game more interesting.

SEE ALSO

Promoting your child's development: ages 5–12   **52–53**

Identifying a child with developmental delay   **196–197**

Creative painting

Cutting sponges into shapes to make stamps can help encourage your child's artistic talents. Wide artist's paintbrushes will be easier for a young child to use than small ones.

USING BOOKS FROM AN EARLY AGE

One of the surest ways to develop your child's intellectual abilities is to introduce her to the pleasure of books. From an early age she will enjoy the experience of being cuddled against you while you look at a simple picture book.

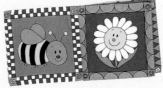

First books for babies are normally wipeable, laminated board books. They feature simple pictures of everyday objects and use bold colours to attract the baby's interest.

By the age of two, she will be able to follow simple stories with bright illustrations. Books with a repeating line or rhyme allow children to take an active part as the story progresses. Pop-up and lift-the-flap books are enjoyed by children throughout this age range.

Preschool children enjoy a whole range of different books – fairy tales, realistic stories, poetry and nonfiction that gives simple information about topics in which they are interested.

Promoting your child's development: ages 5–12

The years between 5 and 12 are childhood proper, when your child begins to show real independence and major stages of development take place.

Starting primary school full-time and beginning secondary school are major transitions for any child. They are both periods when a child has to take responsibility for himself in a new environment and are significant steps toward his becoming independent of you.

At primary school, your child will have to deal with new situations without your direct input; however, if you have provided him with a secure home life, he will probably not find this transition difficult.

Once your child enters secondary school – usually at about 11 years of age – he will spend most of his day there and feel even more removed from home than he did when in primary school, and you will probably have much less involvement.

Musical instruments
Learning how to play an instrument, whether a violin, recorder, guitar or the drums, improves motor skills and teaches cooperation.

Despite some initial nervousness, he should be able to settle down into a completely separate school existence.

As more is expected of children in terms of formal learning and disciplined routines, your child may revert to some babyish habits. You should not remark on them, unless they continue for a long time. If this does happen, consult your child's teacher to discover what could be upsetting him.

Reading and maths

Learning to read is perhaps the most significant intellectual development that your child will achieve during this stage. It is important to remember that children develop at remarkably different rates and a child not reading at the age of six will not necessarily go on to fail as a teenager or adult. Continue to encourage him by looking at books together and don't make too much of a fuss if he is struggling. You should make sure he sees you reading for pleasure yourself. If he has one or two favourite television programmes, try to find books related to them.

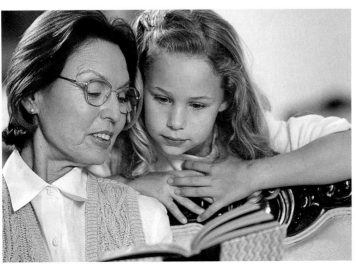

Reading with your child
Although your child, or grandchild, can read by herself, you can still encourage her by allowing her to read to you or by reading to her from a book in which she will recognize most, but not necessarily all, the words.

OVERSTIMULATION

Although most parents worry about too much television, few acknowledge the problem of overstimulation. There is increasing concern that children are encouraged to participate in such a large number of extracurricular activities that they are in danger of "burning out". It is important to allocate time when your child can just relax and be a normal child.

You should only encourage an activity in which your child expresses an interest, and even then wait a while in case the desire to learn piano or dancing is just a whim. Learning new skills involves practice time and most children give up before becoming competent. When you decide to allow your child to try a new skill, encourage him without applying pressure. Low-key activities such as youth clubs are fine – they concentrate on socializing.

Mathematical skills, which are as significant as being able to read, will also be improving. If you are a less-than-confident mathematician yourself, you might consider taking a course to help become aware of what your child is tackling – you may be surprised at how the teaching of this subject has changed.

Understanding life

Abstract ideas will begin to flourish and are often accompanied by questions on life, sex and death. Your answers will depend on your beliefs; however, you must be prepared for your child to become increasingly influenced by his peers and television. Peer pressure comes into its own now, and it is an unwise parent who wages war against his child's friends. Comment little on what his friends say or do, but make it clear you will not be influenced by what other children are allowed and by other parents' rulings. Encouraging friends and getting to know their parents is the best way of providing the support your child needs.

Modern technology

Television and computer games are an ever-growing cause of concern for parents. If you don't want your child to watch television endlessly, you'll have to foster other interests and perhaps even do some activities with him. You should also be seen to spend your free time doing things other than watching televsion.

Many films and programmes made for adults are shown later in the evening to avoid children seeing unsettling scenes. However, some children's cartoons have elements of violence that could be disturbing to certain children. You should use your own judgement to decide what you consider suitable for your child to watch and not be influenced otherwise. You know your child – if he is likely to have nightmares after watching something frightening, you must make the decision to turn the television off.

As children reach their preteen years, they will probably spend time at their friends' houses, as well as at home, playing computer games and on the Internet. Take time to familiarize yourself with the equipment and what they are doing. The games are marked with recommended ages and you should take notice of these. To ensure the television and computer are turned off for a while and that your child gets exercise, encourage him to play a sport or swim.

SEE ALSO
Promoting your child's
development: under 5   **50–51**
Identifying a child with
developmental delay   **196–197**

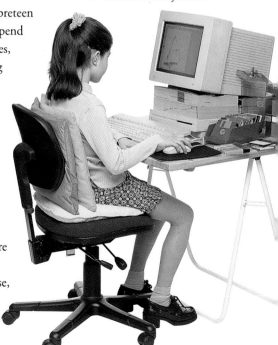

Sitting at a computer
Instruct your child how to sit at a computer properly: her back should be straight and well supported, her feet flat on the ground and she should not have to bend her arms at more than a 45-degree angle to reach the keyboard.

Caring for a sick child

All children are occasionally ill, which will naturally cause you some concern. Fortunately, however, most illnesses are not serious and most children will recover quickly after a few days of rest.

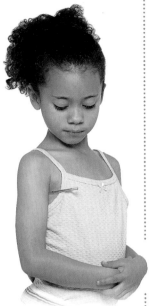

Taking a child's temperature
For a child under seven years old, only use a mercury thermometer by placing it under her armpit. She shouldn't move her arm away for five minutes. (Try sitting a restless child on your lap and holding her arm.)

While she is sick, your child may be more demanding than usual, so you will need to be patient. Being in the same room as you or within speaking distance is less frightening or lonely for a young child. Unless your child wants to go to bed or your doctor advises bed rest, tuck her up on a sofa or armchair with a pillow and cover her with a sheet and light blanket or a duvet. Don't allow your child to become overheated – dress her in light, comfortable clothes such as cotton pyjamas or a short-sleeve cotton shirt and trousers. Wrapping a child up warmly or overheating a room may cause a febrile convulsion in a child who has a fever.

Encourage your child to drink plenty of fluids, and let her choose her favourite one. If she is reluctant to drink, try ice lollies made with real fruit juice or freeze fruit juice in ice cube trays and let her suck the cubes. Or make milk shakes in her choice of flavour. Don't worry if she does not want to eat much. Offer some light foods, such as jelly, or let her choose what she feels like eating. Avoid dairy products if she is congested, because they encourage mucus production.

Taking a temperature

The normal body temperature is 37°C (98.6°F) but this may vary a little. If your child has a fever, her temperature will be over 37.7°C (99.9°F). Fever is the most common symptom in childhood and causes a lot of anxiety. It can occur with a variety of infectious and noninfectious diseases or following vaccination.

Parents can usually tell if a child is feverish simply by touching the forehead, but there may be times when you need to take her temperature. Only take your child's temperature by mouth if she is seven years of age or older. (An armpit reading is 0.6°C/1.1°F lower than one from the mouth.) Before using a mercury thermometer for an older child, shake it until the mercury returns to the bulb, and rinse it in cold water after reading it.

Lowering a temperature

Temperatures below 39°C (102.2°F) are not in themselves thought to be harmful, because they mean that the child is fighting off the infection that caused the

TYPES OF THERMOMETER

The standard mercury thermometer can be difficult to use on a child who fidgets. Other types include the strip thermometer, which is placed across the forehead but does not give an accurate reading, and digital thermometers, which are easy to read. One type of digital thermometer is placed under the tongue or armpit and gives a reading after a few minutes. The best type – and most expensive – is an ear digital thermometer; it gives a reading one second after placing it in the ear canal.

Digital ear thermometer

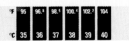

°F	95	96.8	98.6	100.4	102.2	104
°C	35	36	37	38	39	40

Strip thermometer

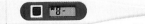

Digital thermometer

fever. If the temperature rises above 39°C (102.2°F) or it rises too quickly, children between six months and five years of age are at risk of having febrile convulsions.

To reduce a high temperature and keep your child comfortable, give plenty of cool, clear fluids. Undress the child to a vest and nappies or panties, and cover her with a sheet. Keep the room cool. Give paracetamol or ibuprofen in the recommended dose for your child's age every four hours. If the temperature is 40–41°C (104–106°F), after taking the above measures, start wiping the child down with a flannel or sponge soaked in tepid water. Cold water should not be used – it causes the blood vessels to contract so less heat will be lost. You should then consult your doctor.

Giving medicines

If the instructions for giving medicine are unclear, ask your doctor or pharmacist for advice. Here are some guidelines:
- Never give your child more than the recommended dose.

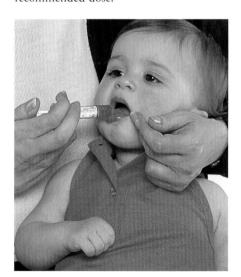

Giving medicine to a baby
For a baby who has not learned how to take food from a spoon, you can give medicine to her with a syringe, available from a chemist.

- Always use a medicine spoon or a liquid medicine measure or syringe.
- If your child is old enough to understand, explain that the medicine will help her to get better.
- Give a favourite drink or some fruit to help take away any unpleasant taste.
- Always finish a course of antibiotics even if your child seems to be better.
- Tell your doctor if your child has a reaction to the medicine.
- Try to use unsweetened medicines whenever you can.
- Make sure you keep all medicines in child-resistant containers and safely out of the reach of your child.
- Never give a reduced dose of adult medicine to a young child.
- Don't give a medicine prescribed for someone else to your child.
- Don't pretend medicines are sweets.
- Never give aspirin to a child under the age of 12, unless under your doctor's supervision – aspirin has been linked to the rare, but serious, condition known as Reye's syndrome.

SEE ALSO

Reye's syndrome and aspirin **63**

Vomiting, diarrhoea
and constipation **96–97**

Febrile convulsions **167**

Keeping baby cool
When your baby is running a fever, dress her in nappies and perhaps a T-shirt or vest to help her cool down – don't bundle her up in layers of clothes.

Using a measuring spoon
An older child can be given medicine with a spoon. You should use the spoon that is supplied with the medicine.

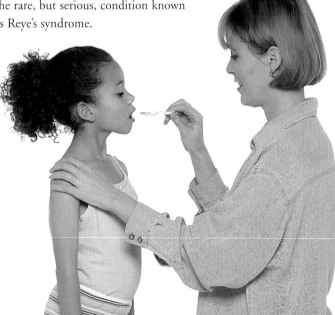

Helping your child in hospital

Sometimes hospital treatment for a child is unavoidable – for an illness or operation, perhaps, or after an accident. You can help make his experience less scary.

WHAT TO PACK

An extended stay in hospital can be made more comfortable for your child and yourself by packing the items listed below.

For your child:
- Two sets of nightclothes
- Comfortable day clothes that are easy to put on
- Toiletries such as soap, skin cream, toothbrush and toothpaste
- Flannel, hand towel and bath towels (unless provided by hospital)
- Comb and hairbrush
- Favourite toy, books and comforter
- Favourite dummy, bottle, cup or beaker.

For you:
- Cool, comfortable clothes
- Nightwear
- Washbag with toiletries
- Something to do (such as books to read, knitting)
- Change or paycard for the telephone
- Simple snacks such as fruit, drinks and biscuits.

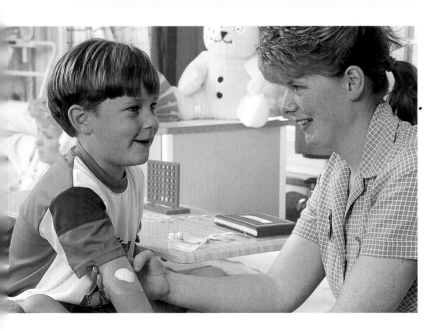

There is a lot you can do to prepare your child for going into hospital and to help ensure his stay is as stress-free as possible. How your child reacts to being in hospital will depend a great deal on his age and personality, the reason for admission and any previous experience of hospitals. If you know in advance that your child will have to go into hospital, try to prepare him as far as possible, depending on his age and level of understanding. Because young children have little idea of time, a day or two in advance is probably best for a toddler.

You can tell a younger child who is ill that he is going into hospital to make him feel better. If he needs an operation, explain, using simple words, what is about to happen. Some children like to know more than others. Answer any questions in a simple but factual way and, most of all, be honest. If your child asks whether something will hurt, it is better to say that it may hurt for a little while, but will not last long and will help to make him better.

Making your child feel at ease

Although going into hospital can be an anxious time for both child and parents, most children's wards are friendly, happy places, staffed by nurses who are specially trained to understand the needs of their young patients.

Before a younger child goes into hospital encouraging him to play doctors and nurses with a toy medical kit or letting him bandage a teddy bear can help. Also read him books with hospital stories or show him pictures of hospital activities. Some hospitals organize informal visits to a ward before admission.

It is important to remember that whenever you are in a hospital, under no circumstances should you use a mobile phone. They can interfere with some of the hospital's monitoring equipment.

Your child in hospital

Most hospitals encourage a parent to stay overnight with a young child. If this is not possible, organize a rota of other relatives and be there for important procedures or times such as bedtime or when he wakes up after an operation. If you have difficulties in visiting your child, such as financial problems, living a long way off or having other children to care for, speak to the hospital social worker.

If you are not able to be with your child all the time, tell the nurse anything extra she needs to know about him. For example, if he has a special word for the potty, bottle or dummy or if there is any food or drink that he dislikes.

Tell the nurses or speak to the doctor if you have any concerns about your child or his treatment. If you and the staff wish, you can carry out some simple procedures such as giving your child his medicine. Sharing in the care of your child by washing, changing and feeding him is also reassuring for him.

Home again

Children coming home from hospital may need time to adjust to normal home life again. A toddler may be clingy and not want to let you out of his sight. An older child may revert to babyish ways. Other siblings may also be jealous or resentful if you have not been there for them. These are all natural reactions and with patience and understanding will usually soon pass.

SEE ALSO
Caring for a sick child 54–55
Jealousy and sulking 176–177
Coping with emergencies 208–219

THINGS TO DO

You can read stories to your child and give him his favourite toys to play with, but play activities may also be provided by trained play staff. For older children there may be a hospital school that he can attend. In addition, depending on your child's age and illness, you may need to provide other activities or think of things for him to do that do not require much concentration.

These could include:

- Simple board games, colouring books or paper and crayons
- A portable cassette player and some tapes of your child's favourite nursery rhymes, pop songs or stories
- Handheld electronic games
- A tray that your child can use for different activities such as assembling simple jigsaws, solving puzzles, using play dough, or playing card games
- Old magazines or catalogues for him to cut up if he is old enough to handle scissors safely.

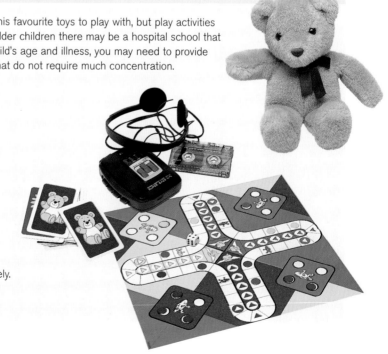

CHAPTER TWO

Health problems and diseases

Only a minority of children will suffer from a chronic or serious life-threatening condition; however, even the healthiest child will occasionally get sick at some stage as she grows up. The majority of children will bounce back from most illnesses quickly, but any illness, no matter how minor it is, can be worrying – especially if you are a first-time parent or if you don't know why your child is feeling unwell.

Understanding the cause of the disease, the treatment available and what you can do to help your child recover as quickly as possible will help you care for your child. Better still, taking preventive measures may help safeguard against the disease occurring in the first place, or stop it from recurring.

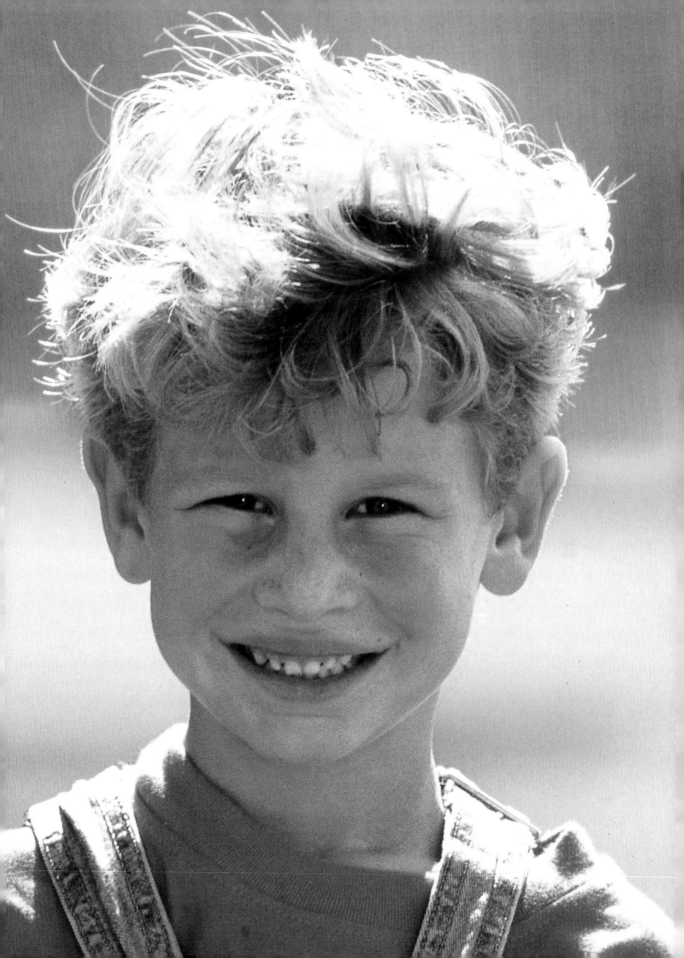

Infectious diseases

A major cause of illness and death used to be infectious diseases. Improvements in health and hygiene, antibiotics and immunization have eliminated some serious infections and greatly reduced the frequency and severity of others.

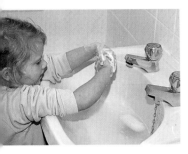

Keeping clean
Teaching your child good hygiene practices, such as washing her hands before eating and after using the toilet, can prevent infection.

Playmates
Children are ill more often when they first have long sessions of interaction with other children – this is normal. They build up immunity and have fewer bouts of illness as they get older.

Infections are still a major cause of illness in children, and they range from a mild cold to a life-threatening illness such as meningitis. They occur when the body has been invaded by disease-causing microorganisms (living creatures that are too tiny to be seen by the naked eye). The most common ones, which cause the majority of infections, are viruses and bacteria. Other microorganisms are fungi and protozoa (microscopic animals). Once microorganisms enter the body they establish themselves and multiply.

Infectious diseases are often called communicable diseases, which means they can be spread from person to person. An infection may enter the body in several ways. For example, by breathing in air containing tiny droplets of infected mucus from an infected person's sneeze; through a cut or wound in the skin; or through infected food or drink. They may affect just one part of the body, such as the throat, or most of the body such as in septicaemia (blood poisoning).

Viruses

Many common diseases are caused by viruses. It may be a mild infection, such as a cold, or a life-threatening disease such as AIDS. Other diseases caused by viruses include chickenpox, rubella and mumps. Viruses also cause 80 to 90 percent of respiratory infections, which are the most common illnesses in childhood. Viruses can only grow inside another living cell, where they reproduce. They are not killed by antibiotics, so your doctor will not prescribe them.

Once a child has been infected with a viral disease, he is usually immune for life. In the cases of colds, however, about 200 "cold-causing viruses" have been identified. Infection from one type of cold virus does not make a child immune to other types, so parents often complain that their child is "never free from a cold". Until they build up resistance to cold viruses, preschool children may have four to eight episodes of coughs and colds a year, and between seven and nine infections a year in the early school years.

Bacteria

Single-celled living microorganisms, bacteria can live outside the body, for example, in the soil. Not all bacteria cause disease or are harmful. In fact, some

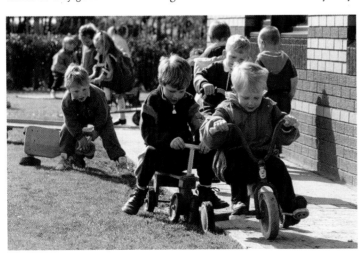

bacteria, known as natural flora, live in the mouth, nose, intestines and on the skin, where they may prevent the growth of other, harmful bacteria.

Bacteria can cause an enormous range of infections, such as boils, meningitis, diphtheria and tetanus. Some bacteria may be killed by antibiotics or germicides.

How the body defends itself

The body has a complex defence system – the immune system. It consists of a collection of specialized cells, such as white blood cells (for example, lympho-cytes) and antibodies, which work together to protect the body or give immunity from invasion by harmful microorganisms such as bacteria and viruses. Some white blood cells develop a memory of the microorganism, so if the same invader attacks again, they are able to get rid of it before it can make the person ill. This is why we get diseases such as chickenpox or measles only once; it is also how immunization works.

Babies are born with some antibodies from their mothers, which gives them immunity to certain diseases for a short period after birth. Vaccinations also provide immunity to certain diseases.

SEE ALSO

Immunization   **20–21**

Allergies and hay fever   **78**

Vomiting, diarrhoea
and constipation   **96–97**

The immune system

A number of barriers in the human body provide the first line of defence against many invading organisms.

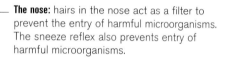

The eyes: the tears contain an enzyme called lysozyme that destroys bacteria.

The mouth: saliva contains enzymes and other substances that destroy bacteria.

Stomach and intestines: acid inside the stomach destroys harmful microorganisms. In the lower intestines, friendly bacteria, or natural flora, help control harmful bacteria. Vomiting and diarrhoea are also methods in which the stomach and intestines rapidly remove toxic substances.

The nose: hairs in the nose act as a filter to prevent the entry of harmful microorganisms. The sneeze reflex also prevents entry of harmful microorganisms.

Respiratory tract: the lining of the bronchioles (see pp.74–75) is covered with cells that contain cilia (fine hairs) and mucus-secreting cells. Microorganisms are trapped by the mucus and swept by the cilia to the bronchi, where they are expelled by coughing.

Genito-urinary system: the vagina and urethra contain natural flora and are protected by mucus.

The skin: undamaged skin acts as a primary barrier against infection. The sebaceous glands (see pp.100–101) secrete chemicals that are toxic to many bacteria. The constant shedding of the outermost cells of the skin also dislodges microorganisms.

Glandular fever

Also known as infectious mono-nucleosis, this illness is caused by a herpes virus called the Epstein-Barr virus. Because it is transmitted by close contact with saliva, it is sometimes called "the kissing disease". It is most common in adolescents and young adults, but it occasionally affects younger children.

The main symptoms are tiredness, fever, headache, sore throat and a generalized enlargement of the lymph nodes. These may be felt as rubbery swellings in the neck, armpits and throat. The spleen is also enlarged and there may be jaundice. Sometimes there is difficulty in breathing and chest pain. In 5 to 10 percent of cases, there may be a widespread pink rash. Rarely, the spleen may rupture, causing blood loss and shock – call the doctor immediately if there is sudden abdominal pain or other significant symptoms. Younger children may have no symptoms, or the symptoms may be nonspecific such as fever and malaise. Diagnosis is confirmed by blood tests.

There is no treatment, but allow the child to rest when he wants. The infection may persist for one to three months. There is full recovery, but fatigue may last for several months.

Mumps

A type of viral infection, mumps mainly affects children over the age of two. In some cases, the symptoms may be so mild as to go unnoticed, but the infection can cause complications.

Mumps is spread by direct contact with saliva or airborne droplets (see p.60). The incubation period (the time from exposure until the symptoms appear) is 15 to 24 days. The most recognizable symptom is swelling of the glands along the jaw. There may be swelling in one gland, then a day or two later, the opposite gland may also swell.

The child may have pain or earache when chewing or swallowing and be unwell with a headache and fever. He is infectious from about six days before the gland swelling until about four days afterward.

Give your child plenty of fluids and soft foods if swallowing is painful. Fruit juice increases saliva and makes the pain worse. Give a non-aspirin painkiller to bring any fever down and help relieve pain. Consult your doctor if your child has a headache with a stiff neck, if he has a persistent earache, if his testicles are swollen or if there is abdominal pain.

Mumps can be prevented by the MMR vaccine between 12 and 15 months of age, with a second dose on starting school.

Complications

A case of mumps can have serious complications, including viral meningitis, encephalitis, deafness (which may be permanent), pancreatitis, oophoritis (inflammation of the ovaries) in females and orchitis (inflammation of the testes) in males. There is no evidence that orchitis causes sterility.

A swollen face

The most recognizable symptom of mumps is the swelling of the parotid salivary glands (the glands that produce saliva) below the ear and along the jaw line.

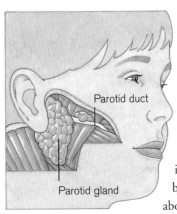

Parotid duct

Parotid gland

Chickenpox

The varicella zoster virus causes chickenpox, a highly infectious disease. It is usually a mild illness in children, but it can have serious complications, especially in those with leukaemia or other immunosuppressing diseases.

Chickenpox is transmitted by infected droplets (see p.60) and by direct contact with fluid from skin lesions or recently infected materials. It usually starts with a mild fever and malaise. This is followed by small, itchy, dark red spots, which appear in crops over three to four days, mainly on the trunk and face. Tiny blisters may appear in the mouth. The spots become blisters (vesicles) and crust over to form scabs. The different stages of the rash – red spots, blisters and scabs – are present at the same time. Rare complications include encephalitis, meningitis and bacterial skin infection.

The incubation period lasts up to three weeks after exposure, and it is infectious from four days before the rash until the last blister is crusted over (usually five to six days after onset of the rash).

Antibiotics are not used to treat chickenpox because it is caused by a virus. Zoster immunoglobulin (ZIG) may be given to prevent chickenpox in a vulnerable child who has been in contact with the disease. In a few countries, such as the United States, a vaccine is given against chickenpox. The antiviral drug acyclovir may be given to treat a vulnerable child who has the disease. Aspirin must never be given to children with chickenpox (see box, above right).

Most adults are immune to chickenpox, but if a pregnant women develops it in the first three months of pregnancy, the foetus is at risk of congenital varicella

REYE'S SYNDROME AND ASPIRIN

A rare disease, Reye's syndrome predominantly affects children and is potentially life threatening. It is almost always preceded by a viral infection such as chickenpox or influenza. Symptoms include uncontrollable vomiting, irrational behaviour or delirium, convulsions and, later, coma. The liver may be enlarged but there is no jaundice.

The cause is not known but there has been a link with the use of aspirin during a viral disease. It is now recommended that aspirin should never be given to children under the age of 12 for any illness.

syndrome. This is rare but includes brain damage, skin scarring, growth retardation and cataracts. Zoster immunoglobulin is given to a pregnant woman who has not had chickenpox and has been in contact with someone who has the disease.

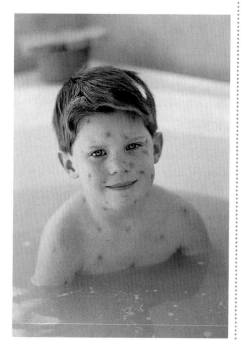

Relieving the itch

The excruciating itch often associated with chickenpox can be eased by applying calamine lotion, or by giving the child a cool bath with bicarbonate of soda added.

Fifth disease

Also known as erythema infectiosum, or slapped cheek syndrome, this infection is caused by the parovirus B19. It is most common in children between the ages of 5 and 15, but it can occur in adults. Complications are rare in children but those with an immune deficiency, such as HIV (see p.73), or chronic blood disorders may become seriously ill.

Fifth disease starts with a mild fever and a nasal discharge. A bright red rash similar to a slap appears on the cheeks about a week later. Over the next two to four days, a red, lacelike rash spreads to the trunk and limbs. This may last for about 10 days. The incubation period is 13 to 18 days and the infection is spread via droplet infection (see p.60) or from a mother to a baby during pregnancy.

Usually no treatment is necessary. Occasionally an older child may have joint pains. Because parovirus B19 temporarily suppresses the production of red blood cells, children with chronic haemolytic anaemia, such as sickle cell anaemia or thalassaemia, may suffer an aplastic crisis (become severely anaemic).

Most pregnant women will be immune to parovirus B19 but rarely, if the woman has the infection, there may be a risk to the foetus. Pregnant women who come into contact with the infection should see their doctor as soon as possible.

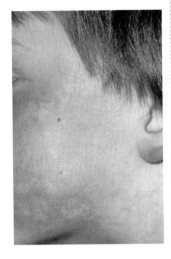

Slapped cheek

The common name is taken from the rash that appears across the child's cheek.

Hand, foot and mouth disease

Although it is a mild infection, hand, foot and mouth disease is contagious and can occur in epidemics. It is caused by the coxsackie virus – not the foot and mouth disease associated with cattle. The disease is common in young children, but it can spread to other family members.

Tiny ulcers or blisters appear on the tongue and inside the cheeks, and small, round or oval, greyish blisters surrounded by redness appear on the palms of the hands and soles of the feet. The child may have a slight fever and be reluctant to eat; otherwise, there are no symptoms. The incubation period is three to five days. The virus also infects the gastrointestinal tract and is present in faeces.

You can relieve the discomfort by giving your child paracetamol and fluids (but avoid fruit juice, which may sting the ulcers). Hand washing may be important in the prevention of the disease, especially after using the toilet.

Typical rash

Small blisters on the palms of the hands and soles of the feet remain contagious until the crusts that form over the blisters and the fluid in them disappear.

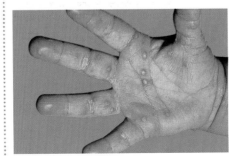

Influenza

This is an acute viral infection of the respiratory tract, which affects all age groups. It is highly contagious and occurs in epidemics, usually in the winter. It is more serious in children who have a chronic medical condition.

SEE ALSO

Caring for a sick child	**54–55**
Infectious diseases	**60–61**
Ear problems	**86–87**
Febrile convulsions	**167**

Popularly called flu, influenza is caused by three types of virus: A, B and C. It is spread by droplets of infected mucus coughed or sneezed into the air. Once a person has had an attack of a particular strain of flu, antibodies are acquired that provide immunity to that strain. However, Type A, which is responsible for most large flu epidemics, is constantly changing or mutating. This means that new strains are produced regularly, resulting in a new epidemic every few years to which people are not immune. Type B, which changes less often, causes less extensive and more localized outbreaks. The illness is not as severe as that of Type A. Type C produces a milder illness and is less common; it provides antibodies for life.

Flu symptoms vary according to the strain, but include a high fever, chills, headache, muscle aches, loss of appetite, tiredness and a dry cough. There may be a sore throat, nausea and weakness. Symptoms appear one to three days after exposure to the virus. In most cases, the acute symptoms last for four or five days, but a cough and tiredness may last longer. Complications in children include otitis media (ear infection) and febrile convulsions in babies and toddlers.

Treatment

Although there is no specific cure for flu, you can help relieve the symptoms. Give a child under 12 years of age a non-aspirin analgesic or painkiller (aspirin has been linked to a serious condition known as Reye's syndrome; see p.63) to reduce the fever and help relieve the aches and pains.

Children with a chronic medical condition such as heart disease, renal disease, diabetes, cancer or asthma are at greatest risk from flu and may require hospitalization (see pp.56–57).

Prevention

An annual influenza vaccine is advisable for children who have chronic medical conditions, including asthma, diabetes mellitus, heart disease and renal failure, and for children with suppressed immune systems or HIV infection. Fit children do not need the vaccine.

As far as possible, you should keep your child away from crowds during a flu epidemic. Children who have flu should be kept away from others.

Recuperating

A child with influenza should be encouraged to drink plenty of fluids. Bed rest isn't essential, but if your child wishes to take a nap, let him – whether in bed or curled up on the sofa.

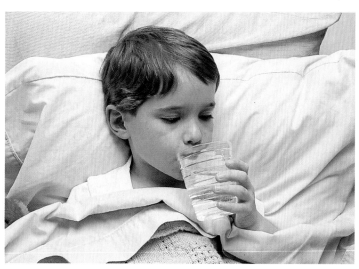

Meningitis

When the membranes, or meninges, that line the brain and spinal cord become inflamed, meningitis is the result. It can occur in any age group – including adults – but the under fives are particularly vulnerable.

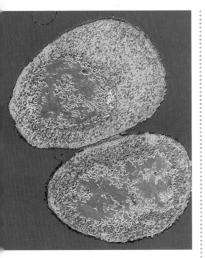

Bacterial meningitis
The bacteria that cause this type of meningitis usually occur in pairs. Here they are shown magnified 28,800 times.

There are several types of meningitis, which can be caused by a viral or bacterial infection. Viral meningitis, the most common type, is rarely serious or life threatening. Bacterial meningitis, however, may be potentially fatal – but if it is diagnosed and treated early, most children will make a full recovery. The symptoms of both types are similar at first, but it is important to distinguish between them to ensure correct treatment.

The incubation period is between 2 and 10 days for bacterial meningitis, and up to three weeks for viral meningitis.

Viral meningitis

This type of meningitis is more common in the winter months, and it may occur as a result of infection from measles, mumps, chickenpox, polio or the cold sore (herpes simplex) virus. Mild cases may even pass unnoticed.

Bacterial meningitis

Although bacterial meningitis is rare, it can be dangerous. There are three main types, which are caused by different organisms: *Haemophilus influenzae* type b (Hib), pneumococcal and meningococcal. All three types occur in children under five years of age. Hib meningitis is now rare because of protection from the Hib vaccine. However, Hib does not protect against other forms of bacterial meningitis or against viral meningitis.

Streptococcus pneumoniae meningitis is the second most common type of bacterial meningitis. It may be transmitted from the respiratory tract into the bloodstream, or can be the result of a fractured skull or an infection in the middle ear.

Meningococcal meningitis is the most common form of bacterial meningitis. One person in 10 carries the bacteria at the back of the throat with no ill effects. Only rarely do they cause illness. Meningococci can be divided into groups

SIGNS OF MENINGITIS

With meningitis or septicaemia, any of these symptoms may be present and can appear in any order. They may not all be present at the same time, and some may not appear at all.

Symptoms of meningitis in babies include:

- A high-pitched, shrill or moaning cry
- Refusing to feed; vomiting
- A blank or staring expression
- Being difficult to wake up or being lethargic
- Pale, blotchy skin
- Dislike of being handled
- Fever, which may be accompanied by cold hands and feet
- Neck retraction with arching of back or floppy body
- A tense or bulging fontanelle (the soft spot on top of the head)
- Rash of red-purple spots or bruises that does not fade when pressed (see opposite).

Symptoms of meningitis in older children include:

- Vomiting
- Severe headache
- High temperature; fever
- Neck stiffness
- Joint pains
- Drowsiness or confusion
- Dislike of bright lights
- Rash of red-purple spots or bruises that does not fade when pressed (see opposite).

A, B and C. Those mostly causing illness in Great Britain belong to groups B and C. Group B is more common in children under two years of age, and group C in young people 14 to 18 years old. Parental smoking is a risk factor for a child's contracting meningococcal meningitis.

Meningococcal disease is the medical name for meningococcal meningitis and septicaemia (blood poisoning). Septicaemia is the more serious of the two illnesses. The disease is most common in the winter months.

Symptoms

Sometimes it can be difficult to tell what type of illness is making your baby or child unwell. In the early stages some of the symptoms of meningitis, such as refusing a feed, vomiting, a rash or a fever (see box, opposite), are also signs of other less serious illnesses. However, a child with bacterial meningitis or septicaemia may become seriously ill extremely quickly. If you have any doubts, you should speak to your doctor.

With meningococcal meningitis or septicaemia, a rash may appear anywhere on the skin; however, the rash is not present in all cases of meningitis. If it is present and does not change colour after the glass tumbler test (see below), it is important to seek medical help immediately. Contact your doctor or take your child directly to the nearest Accident and Emergency Department.

Treatment

Early treatment of meningococcal meningitis with antibiotics can save your child's life. The doctor will give him an injection of benzyl penicillin to halt it before it becomes life threatening, and he'll admit your child to hospital. The main complication caused by bacterial meningitis in children is deafness. Approximately 10 percent of cases are fatal. Full recovery may take weeks or months.

As a preventive measure, an antibiotic will be given to anybody who has been in close contact with a person who has meningococcal disease. In some countries, all children should be immunized against Group C meningococcus by the 21st century, and close contacts of people with group C meningoccoccal disease may be offered the vaccine. However, there is no specific treatment for viral meningitis.

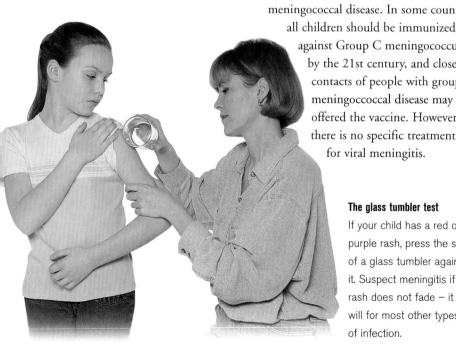

The glass tumbler test
If your child has a red or purple rash, press the side of a glass tumbler against it. Suspect meningitis if the rash does not fade – it will for most other types of infection.

SEE ALSO
Immunization 20–21
Helping your child in hospital 56–57
Infectious diseases 60–61

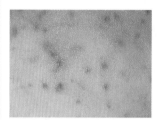
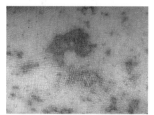

Meningitis rash
The rash may start as a cluster of tiny blood spots that resemble pin pricks (top). In an advanced stage the rash may look like reddish purple blotches or bruises (bottom).

Measles

This highly infectious viral disease occurs mostly in childhood. Babies usually have a natural immunity from their mothers in the first six to eight months of life, and immunization thereafter has reduced the number of cases.

For children who catch measles, it remains a dangerous disease, with 1 child in 15 developing complications. Measles is caused by the rubeola virus. It is spread by droplet infection (see p.60) and the first symptoms appear 7 to 20 days after exposure to the virus. Symptoms are similar to those of a bad cold, with malaise, a runny nose, a high fever, sore and red watery eyes and a cough.

The early symptoms last three to four days, after which a rash of brownish pink spots appears behind the ears. The child will be miserable and may be ill before the rash appears and while it is developing. One or two days before the rash, Koplik's spots – small white spots similar to grains of salt – may be seen inside the mouth. They are a useful way to identify the onset of measles. Some children may also have swollen lymph glands or become sensitive to light.

Treatment

Call your doctor if you suspect your child has measles. Antibiotics may be prescribed, but only for a secondary bacterial infection. You should allow your child rest, keep her cool and give plenty of clear fluids and a non-aspirin fever-reducing medicine to help lower any temperature.

If a child has not received the MMR vaccine, it can be given at any age to protect her during an outbreak – however, it should be given within three days of exposure. Rarely, some children, such as those receiving immunosuppressive treatment, should not be given the vaccine; however, immunoglobulin can be given to protect her if she has been exposed to measles.

Measles rash

The rash spreads down from the face to the neck, trunk and limbs, usually over three days, and fades in the same order that it appeared. The spots may spread so much that they merge to form blotches.

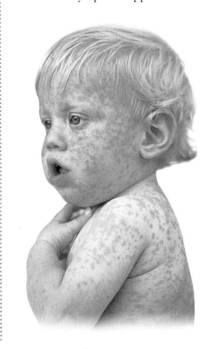

COMPLICATIONS

- Complications may include pneumonia, bronchitis (see p.81), otitis media (see pp.86–87) and febrile convulsions (see p.167).
- Encephalitis, a potentially life-threatening inflammation of the brain cells (see p.166), occurs in 1 in 5,000 cases.
- Children with a chronic medical condition, such as cystic fibrosis (see p.148), heart disease (see p.118), kidney disease (see p.162), or Down's syndrome (see pp.142–143), are at particular risk of developing complications from measles.

Molluscum contagiosum

This superficial skin infection is caused by one of the pox viruses. Firm, flesh-coloured bumps, which are approximately 2–5 mm ($\frac{1}{10}$–$\frac{1}{5}$ in) in diameter, appear on the skin of both children and adults. They are a type of wart and are sometimes known as water warts. The doughnut-shaped bumps have a sunken centre containing a white waxy substance. They can appear anywhere on the body, including the buttocks and genital area (however, bumps in the genital area are seen more often in adults). The bumps may appear alone or in clusters; they may look unsightly, but they are not painful or tender – but they may itch.

The infection is spread on the skin by autoinoculation – that is, by touching or scratching an infected lesion and transferring the virus when a new area of skin is touched with the infected hand. It may be spread to other people by close physical contact or by indirect contact such as sharing towels or in a public swimming pool.

Removing the bumps

Treatment is not usually necessary, but it may be done for cosmetic reasons or to prevent the infection from spreading. There are a number of treatments available, but they can be painful. They include cryosurgery, which involves freezing the individual bumps with liquid nitrogen; curettage, in which the bumps are scraped to remove the centres; laser therapy; and puncturing the bumps to touch the centre with a sharpened wooden orange stick that has been dipped in phenol.

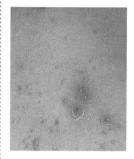

Molluscum rash

The bumps may linger for nine months or more before they suddenly disappear; normally, the rash is not red.

Roseola infantum

The virus known as the human herpes virus 6 is responsible for causing roseola infantum. This is a common, but mild illness, which usually appears in the spring or summer. About one child in three will come down with it. Roseola infantum is also known as exanthem subitum (a medical term that means "sudden rash") and sixth disease.

The infection usually affects children between the ages of six months and three years. There is a sudden onset of a high fever of 39.5–41°C (103–106°F), which lasts for about four days. The child may have swollen glands or be irritable, but may otherwise be well. In some cases the high fever may cause febrile convulsions.

As the temperature returns to normal, the roseola rash appears on the chest, stomach and back, then spreads to the arms and neck. It also appears on the thighs and buttocks. The rash usually lasts from 24 to 48 hours.

Lowering the fever

The main treatment is to reduce your child's temperature to avoid the possibility of a convulsion. Keep your child cool and give her plenty of fluids. Your doctor may also advise giving a non-aspirin medicine to reduce the high temperature. Tepid sponging may be necessary to help reduce the fever. (Antibiotics cannot be used to treat the condition.)

Sudden rash

The rose-coloured rash has flat spots, which turn white when you touch them.

Pertussis

Severe bouts of coughing and choking are the most recognizable signs of pertussis, or whooping cough. This serious, highly contagious infection affects children and adults, but it is more dangerous in young children.

Relentless cough

The bouts of coughing that end in a high-pitched whoop as the child draws in a breath of air gave whooping cough its name.

The bordetella pertussis bacteria causes pertussis. It is spread through airborne droplets when an infected person sneezes, coughs or talks (see p.60). The symptoms appear 7 to 14 days after exposure to the bacteria. At first, they may resemble a cough and cold, with a fever and runny nose. After one or two weeks, the cough changes to repeated bouts of severe coughing in the same breath, which may last for over a minute. During the attack the child may turn blue due to lack of air. Usually, the cough ends in a whooping noise, but this does not always happen in young infants. The coughing bouts are most persistent during the night.

Vomiting can occur during the spells of coughing, because the child may choke on the mucus. This may result in dehydration and weight loss. After the severe bouts of coughing and vomiting cease, a cough may persist for up to three months.

The infection may last for several weeks, and the disease may leave your child debilitated for several months afterward. Possible complications include ear infections (see pp.86–87), pneumonia, bronchitis (see p.81), febrile convulsions (see p.167) and brain damage.

PREVENTION

The pertussis vaccine is usually given as part of the DPT childhood vaccination programme, but there is no upper age limit for the vaccine. If your child has only had the DT vaccine, an acellular pertussis vaccine (APV) course can be given.

Preventive antibiotics may be prescribed for children who have not had the vaccine if another family member in the house has pertussis. You should consult your doctor.

Severe complications and, potentially, death are more common in children under six months old.

Helping your child recuperate

Consult your doctor immediately if you think your child has whooping cough. Although there is no treatment to reduce the duration of the illness, the doctor can prescribe an antibiotic to reduce the period of infectivity, normally for about three weeks after the coughing starts.

Ensure that your child has plenty of fluids. Give him frequent small meals of noncrumbly food, preferably after a bout of coughing or vomiting. Babies may need to be admitted to a hospital.

It is important that you do not expose your child to irritants, such as cigarette smoke or fumes from aerosol sprays or cleaning materials – these can trigger bouts of coughing.

Scarlet fever

A strain of streptococcus bacteria causes the infection known as scarlet fever. In the past, it was a dangerous disease, but treatment with antibiotics means it has ceased to be a serious infection.

Scarlet fever is spread by droplets coughed or sneezed into the air (see p.60) and usually starts with a sore throat, headache and a fever. This is followed by a red rash, which is caused by a toxin produced by the streptococcus bacteria. Although the face is flushed, the area around the mouth remains pale. At first, the tongue may have a white coating with red spots. Later, the coating peels off to reveal a bright red tongue, which is known as a strawberry tongue.

The doctor may diagnose scarlet fever from the signs and symptoms, or he may take a throat swab to grow the bacteria in the laboratory to confirm a streptococcal infection. Antibiotics will then be given to help prevent any risk of complications from streptococci such as rheumatic disease. The child should have plenty of fluids and be given a non-aspirin medication for the sore throat and to reduce the fever.

Scarlet fever rash

The rash starts as tiny red bumps, usually on the neck and face, then spreads to the rest of the body.

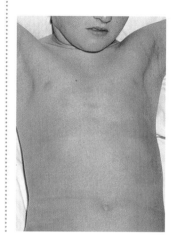

Rubella

Also referred to as German measles, rubella is a viral infection that is most common in children between the ages of four and nine who have not had the rubella immunization.

Symptoms include a mild fever for one or two days, and swollen glands behind the ears, followed by a rash of tiny, pink, slightly raised spots. There may also be swollen glands in other parts of the body, conjunctivitis, a sore throat and headache, and, sometimes, pain and swelling in the joints. The child will be infectious from one week before the onset of the rash until four days afterward.

Usually, the disease is not serious in children, but rubella infection in a woman who is pregnant may cause a serious condition known as congenital rubella syndrome in the unborn child. If exposed to the virus during the first 12 weeks of pregnancy, 80 percent of babies are affected; the rate of infection falls in the following 10 weeks. Babies who are infected may be born with brain damage, deafness, blindness, heart disease, growth retardation or other serious problems.

Treatment

To reduce any fever or discomfort, give a non-aspirin medicine such as paracetamol. If your child develops a high temperature, a severe headache, is drowsy or otherwise appears ill, contact the doctor.

Infected children should be kept away from pregnant women. Before conceiving, all women should have a blood test to confirm they are immune to rubella. If they are not, they should be immunized before becoming pregnant.

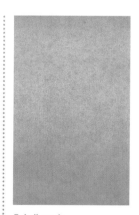

Rubella rash

The rash first appears behind the ears or on the face, then spreads to the rest of the body.

Hepatitis

The word hepatitis means an inflammation of the liver. It is most commonly caused by one of three viruses: hepatitis A, B or C. The severity and long-term effects depend on the type of virus.

Viral hepatitis is a contagious disease, but the viruses spread in different ways. About 40 percent of the population of western Europe have had hepatitis A. A much smaller percentage of the population has hepatitis B, also known as serum hepatitis, and hepatitis C. Some people with the B and C forms do not know they have it because they did not have symptoms; however, they are often carriers and can spread it to others.

Most children with hepatitis A have no symptoms or only mild symptoms such as fever, nausea, vomiting, diarrhoea, loss of appetite, abdominal pain and tiredness. After a week or so, jaundice may develop, with yellowing of the skin and whites of eyes, dark urine and pale- or clay-coloured stools. Children recover within a month.

The symptoms for hepatitis B and C are similar, but they may be more severe – or there may be none at all. There may be chronic liver disease, which will require monitoring by a specialist. A child with hepatitis B may also develop joint pains and a rash.

TYPES OF HEPATITIS

Virus type	How it spreads	Treatment and prevention
Hepatitis A	The hepatitis A virus (HAV) lives in the faeces of infected people. The infection is caught when it is passed into the body through the mouth if the hands, water, utensils or food have been contaminated with the infected faeces.	Encourage good hygiene such as washing hands after using the toilet and before eating. If travelling to areas where sanitation or hygiene is poor, you should first have a hepatitis A vaccine.
Hepatitis B	The hepatitis B virus (HBV) is spread through infected body fluids, particularly blood. HBV-infected mothers may pass the infection on to the baby during or soon after birth. Children should not share toothbrushes, a possible route of transmission.	A nourishing diet is advised for the first several months. Babies born to mothers who have had hepatitis B during pregnancy or who are carriers of the virus should be given immunoglobulin and a course of four vaccines, which must be completed to be effective.
Hepatitis C	Hepatitis C was spread through unscreened blood products and blood transfusions; blood screening has made this route of transmission rare. It can be spread from an infected mother to a baby during pregnancy, but this is also rare. Children should not share toothbrushes, a route of transmission.	A nourishing diet is advised. There is no vaccine against hepatitis C. If the baby is infected, she should be referred to a specialist paediatric unit, where she will be closely monitored. Sometimes a course of treatment with interferon may be recommended.

HIV (AIDS)

The human immunodeficiency virus (HIV), which may cause acquired immune deficiency syndrome (AIDS), is a retrovirus. Mothers who don't know that they are infected can sometimes pass the virus to their babies during birth.

This retrovirus attaches itself to the T-cell lymphocytes (a type of white blood cell), which are crucial to the immune system. The number of healthy T-cells decreases and seriously affects the body's ability to fight infection. As the HIV spreads, the immune system is destroyed and the person develops AIDS.

The HIV virus is carried in blood, saliva and seminal and vaginal fluids. The main way that children acquire the infection is from mother to child transmission – in the uterus, during delivery or during breastfeeding. The risk from contaminated blood products is rare.

Children with HIV infection may fail to thrive or have poor weight gain; they may also suffer from frequent infections such as fungal infections (for example thrush), recurrent bacterial infections, respiratory infections, diarrhoea and viral infections. The main cause of illness and death in infected infants is PCP (pneumonia) in the first months of life.

Treatment

The current progression to AIDS after the initial infection is about 11 years. With advances in drug therapy, survival is likely to improve in the future. Drugs to treat people with HIV are called antiretrovirals. There are three classes of drugs available, but some may not be licensed to treat children in all countries. They are nucleoside analogue reverse transcriptase inhibitors (NRTIs), protease inhibitors and nonnucleoside reverse transcriptase inhibitors (NNRTIs). Because these work in different ways, a combination of drugs may be given.

Preventing mother to child transmission will have the biggest impact on reducing AIDS in children. It is recommended that all pregnant women should be offered HIV testing. If it is discovered that a pregnant woman is HIV positive, steps can be taken to reduce the risk of HIV being passed to the infant by:
● Drug therapy during pregnancy and in early infancy.
● Caesarean section, which is safer for the baby than a vaginal delivery.
● Avoidance of breastfeeding.
● Protecting the baby from infections with preventive medication.

HELPING A CHILD WHO HAS AIDS

Because some drugs have side effects or are difficult to take, children may be reluctant to take them. It is vitally important that the drugs are administered as instructed and at the precise time stated. If doses are missed, the virus may become resistant to the drugs.

In many health districts there are specific services for HIV-infected children and their families. There are also charitable organizations that can give information and support.

There is no risk of a child transmitting HIV to others through everyday social contact such as sharing cutlery or crockery, or using a toilet. An infected child should not be excluded from school or other normal social contact. The main risk is posed to the HIV-infected child, who can develop complications from contracting another disease, particularly measles, chickenpox or herpes. The childhood immunization schedule may differ slightly – your doctor can give further advice about the appropriate schedule for your child.

Knowing the risks
An HIV child can play with others without risk to them – the only risk is to the HIV child.

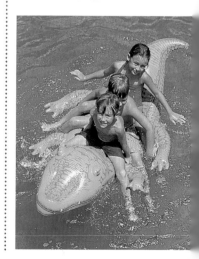

The lungs and respiration

Oxygen is vital for life – in fact, irreparable damage is caused if the body is without it for more than about four minutes. This means that it is extremely important that the respiratory system works efficiently.

The respiratory system
The mouth, nose and throat form the upper respiratory system. The lower respiratory system consists of the trachea, lungs, bronchi, bronchioles and alveoli.

Every cell in the human body needs oxygen to produce energy. However, as energy is released, the poisonous gas carbon dioxide is produced, and this must be removed from the body to prevent fatal levels of the gas building up. The respiratory system exchanges the oxygen in the air that is breathed in with the carbon dioxide in the blood, and the carbon dioxide is expelled during exhalation.

Breathing in and out
The first step in the exchange of gases is to take air – and, therefore, oxygen – into the lungs. These are two spongy bags encased by the ribs and connected to the nose and throat by the airway called the trachea. To draw air into them, the diaphragm – a dome-shaped muscle that runs across the base of the lungs – contracts. This increases the volume of the lungs, which is further increased by an upward and outward swing of the ribs as the rib and chest wall muscles contract. As the volume in the lungs is increased, the pressure of the air in them is reduced, and air is drawn in to equalize it.

The air breathed in travels through the nose and mouth, the pharynx and the larynx – the upper respiratory tract. It enters the trachea, the first part of the lower respiratory tract. This divides into two smaller tubes – the left and right bronchi – and, as the air travels deeper, the tubes continue to subdivide and become smaller, like the branches of a tree – in fact, the system is called the bronchial tree. The most delicate tubes are known as bronchioles. Each one leads to an alveolar duct, from which 30 tiny pouches called alveoli open out.

The millions of alveoli in the lungs are covered with a thin film of water. The oxygen in the alveoli dissolves into this film and is then in direct contact with the alveolar wall, which is only one cell thick. On the other side of the wall is a network

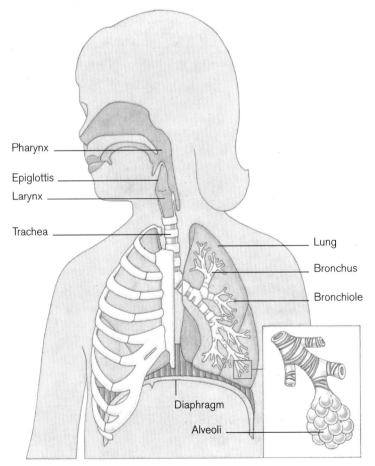

Pharynx

Epiglottis

Larynx

Trachea

Lung

Bronchus

Bronchiole

Diaphragm

Alveoli

of tiny blood vessels, or capillaries. Arterioles deliver to them blood low in oxygen and rich in carbon dioxide, which has travelled around the body before being pumped by the heart to the lungs for replenishment; and venules transport reoxygenated blood back to the heart. The oxygen in the watery film diffuses across the alveolar wall and capillary wall. At the same time, carbon dioxide diffuses from the blood into the watery film on the surface of the alveolus, and eventually into the air in the lungs.

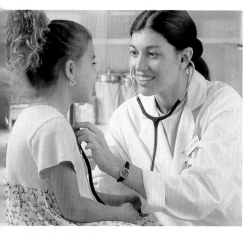

Listening to the lungs
If a child has a suspected chest problem, a doctor or nurse may listen to the lungs with a stethoscope to help determine how well they are functioning.

Finally, the diaphragm and the muscles of the chest wall and ribs relax. This allows the lungs' natural elastic recoil to force air out, and the breath is exhaled.

Because no conscious effort is required to breathe – although it can be put under conscious control if necessary – a control system that works automatically is required. This is provided by a group of nerve cells in the brain called the respiratory centre. Here, information is monitored from chemoreceptors that measure oxygen and carbon dioxide levels

in the arteries; from stretch receptors in the lungs; and from baroreceptors, which measure blood pressure. Having assessed the information, the centre sends signals to the muscles used in breathing, directing them to work harder or less hard. For example, they will work harder when a child runs and less hard when he is asleep.

Protective measures

The airways and lungs contain a series of defences to prevent foreign bodies and disease-causing organisms from entering them. The hairs in the nostrils trap large particles, while the mucous membranes of both the mouth and nose trap bacteria. Tiny hairs, cilia, sweep dust toward the throat, where it is swallowed. The tonsils and adenoids at the back of the mouth produce white cells to destroy bacteria. Further down, the airways are lined with more cilia, which trap foreign bodies and bacteria and sweep them along until they trigger a cough reflex and are expelled.

A child's breathing

When in the uterus, a baby's lungs are not needed and are collapsed until birth. The lungs expand the first time a baby takes in a breath of air. A newborn's breathing is usually irregular, shallow and difficult to hear because his lungs are weak and need time to strengthen. All babies make strange sounds when breathing – this is no cause for concern.

Children often get common colds (see p.80), from which they usually recover quickly, and more children are developing asthma (see pp.76–77), which requires treatment. If something goes seriously wrong with your child's breathing – for example, it is laboured, with his ribs rising sharply each time he breathes in (his lips may also turn blue) – he needs immediate emergency treatment.

SEE ALSO
Infectious diseases   **60–61**
Tonsillitis and pharyngitis   **83**
Heart, blood and
circulation   **114–115**

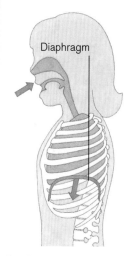

Breathing in
Air enters the lungs as the diaphragm and chest muscles contract to lift the ribcage.

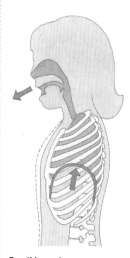

Breathing out
When the diaphragm and the chest muscles relax, the ribcage falls and air is exhaled.

Asthma

The incidence of asthma seems to be increasing. It is estimated that asthma affects 5 percent of people in the world population, and it affects at least 10 percent of children by the time they are the age of 10.

Although the number of asthma sufferers continues to grow, with proper treatment and adequate training asthmatics can learn to live normal lives. Asthma is not a specific disease but a set of symptoms that can be triggered by any of a variety of factors. The condition may have a genetic basis, because it appears to run in families, and involves an allergic response in which antibodies are produced to combat inhaled allergens. Sufferers are often susceptible to other allergies, such as hay fever, and to eczema.

Asthma cannot usually be diagnosed until the age of two, but it may be present earlier; the most common age of onset is seven. Twice as many boys are affected as girls, but in half of all cases – but less often in girls than boys – asthma dies out in early adulthood or attacks become less severe.

The mechanism

The allergic response to inhaled allergens causes the muscles in the walls of the bronchioles to contract, reducing the flow of air and, therefore, oxygen to the alveoli. The bronchiole walls also become inflamed as a result of the allergic response; at the same time, certain glands secrete too much mucus, clogging the airways. Both factors further reduce the flow of air, and oxygen levels in the blood become dangerously reduced, while levels of carbon dioxide rise. The results can be extremely serious, and without treatment an asthma attack can occasionally be fatal.

Most children have only a mild degree of asthma, but there is always the risk that one day a child who has previously had minor attacks will have a major one. It is, therefore, important to seek medical advice as soon as you suspect that a child is asthmatic. Symptoms of an attack include, in order of severity:
- A persistent cough
- Wheezing
- Laboured breathing – the abdomen may be sucked in as attempts are made to take a breath
- Anxiety and panic as the child feels that she is suffocating
- A blue tinge to the lips, indicating oxygen starvation.

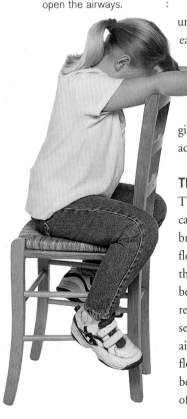

Opening the airways
Difficulty in breathing can be alleviated if your child straddles a chair with her arms over its back and her head resting on her arms. This position helps to expand her chest and open the airways.

WHAT TRIGGERS AN ATTACK

The allergens most often implicated in triggering an attack are pollen, flakes of animal skin and hair, mould spores, certain foods – depending on the individual – and the house dust mite.

Various irritants may set off an attack by stimulating receptors in the bronchioles that contract the muscles, but without there being an allergic response, or production of histamine. Examples include emotional or physical stress, viral infections such as a cold or bronchiolitis (see pp.80–81), diesel fumes, smoke, perfumes, paint and – often with exercise – cold air.

Diagnosis and treatment

Your doctor will test and monitor your child's asthma by using a peak expiratory flow (PEF) meter. The child blows into this simple device as hard as she can and an indicator shows how much air is expelled from her lungs, which indicates how open the airways are. Many asthma sufferers check their PEF daily to see if an attack is likely; the level of air expelled often falls a few days before an attack.

Some types of PEF meter are fitted with a "windmill trainer" for young children to use. It has sails that are turned as air is forced out of the lungs. The amount of pressure required to turn the sails can be adjusted, giving the child a visual guide to improve her breathing techniques.

As the first line of defence against an asthma attack, your doctor is likely to prescribe bronchodilator drugs, which widen the bronchioles. The drugs are usually sprayed into the throat by means of a refillable inhaler, although other methods can be used. If bronchodilators are not effective enough, steroid drugs may be inhaled, or, in more serious cases, given in tablet form; however, steroids in large doses over a long period may have side effects such as suppression of growth.

In a severe attack, large doses of bronchodilators may be required; they are normally given in hospital. Your doctor may refer your child to a phsyiotherapist to learn breathing techniques. She will teach your child how to control her breathing to keep it calm during an attack.

Your child may have to get into the habit of using medication on a daily basis. If your child has been prescribed medication for an attack, it should be used as soon as one starts. If she has no medication, or it seems ineffective, you should call the emergency services as soon as her breathing becomes laboured.

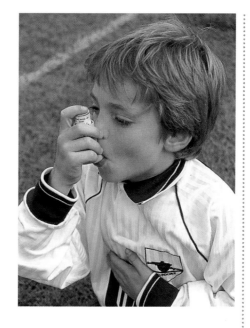

Prevention

The most effective way of preventing an asthma attack is for your child to avoid all contact with the allergen – or allergens – and irritants responsible for triggering an attack. It can be difficult to establish what these are, but to find out what she should avoid, keep a diary of her attacks and the situations in which they occur so you can identify correlations between an attack and changes in her environment.

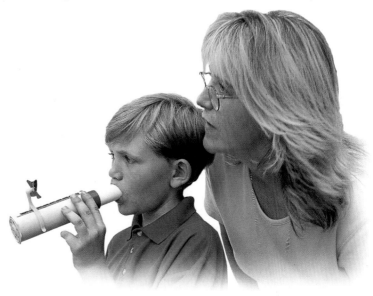

SEE ALSO
The lungs and respiration **74–75**
Allergies and hay fever **78–79**
Food allergies and intolerances **98–99**

Getting fast relief
An inhaler containing bronchodilator drugs can give instant relief. Your child will have to learn how to use it himself – it is important that he learns to use it properly.

Using a peak flow meter
By using a peak flow meter to measure the amount of air your child expels from his lungs, you may be able to predict when an asthma attack is likely.

Allergies and hay fever

Also known as allergic rhinitis, hay fever is one type of allergy that is estimated to affect about one in every six children by the time they become teenagers – and its incidence is increasing.

Hay fever is probably the most common of all allergies, although it rarely affects children until the age of five. This condition tends to run in families, and between 40 and 60 percent of children who suffer from eczema develop hay fever later on. Only children or eldest children have a 75 percent higher risk of developing it. Hay fever attacks generally become less severe as a child grows older and often stop completely.

To fight off infections, the body contains large numbers of antibodies that recognize potentially harmful foreign substances called antigens. When an antibody encounters its antigen, it latches on to it and acts as a marker for defensive cells that can destroy it. Some of these markers, known as IgE antibodies, attract special immune cells that are fast-acting and release powerful chemicals such as histamine.

In hay fever, as in other allergies, a harmless substance is identified as an antigen; these substances are known as allergens. People susceptible to allergies have higher levels of IgE markers in their bodies, so more special cells respond to the allergens and more histamine is released. The next time the allergens are encountered, even more histamine is released because more antibodies have been produced ready to fight it – this process is known as sensitization.

Symptoms

As the body starts to react to the presence of an allergen, there is often a tingly, itching feeling in the eyes, nose, mouth and throat. Then the nose and eyes start to run and the child sneezes to flush the allergens out. Next, the histamine takes effect. It irritates and inflames mucous membranes lining the airway and eyes, making them swell. As a result, the nose may become blocked, causing rhinitis (see box, left), and the eyes may be red, watery and itchy. Inflammation may spread to the sinuses, resulting in sinusitis (see box, left), and to the ears; this may cause a feeling of tightness in the ear and lead to glue ear (see pp.86–87). Some hay fever sufferers also suffer from pollen asthma – when hay fever triggers an asthma attack.

RHINITIS AND SINUSITIS

Although rhinitis – an inflammation of the mucous membranes of the nose – can be caused by hay fever, it can also be the result of a viral infection. The nose runs and becomes congested, and treatment is either as for a cold or for hay fever, depending on the cause.

Sinusitis occurs when the sinus cavities in the skull and cheeks become inflamed and clogged with mucus (the photograph below shows inflamed sinuses above the eyes). It may be a symptom of hay fever; however, it may also be a secondary bacterial infection following a viral infection that has affected the upper respiratory tract. Treatment is the same as for the common cold, but antibiotics may also be necessary. Rarely, in severe cases, the sinuses may need to be drained surgically.

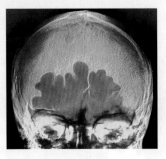

How long the symptoms last and how serious they are depends on the child and on how much exposure there has been to a particular allergen.

Treatment

If you suspect that your child has hay fever, consult your doctor. Bathing irritated eyes relieves discomfort, but drugs may be needed, and there is also the risk that pollen asthma may develop. The first drugs to be tried are usually antihistamine sprays or tablets (which can often be bought without a prescription) and sympathomimetic nose drops. If these are ineffective, stronger corticosteroid drugs may be necessary, but they can have serious side effects when used at high doses over a long period of time.

The most effective form of long-term treatment is prevention. Identify the allergen responsible for your child's hay fever by keeping a diary of attacks. (Your doctor may arrange for common allergens to be tested on your child's skin to help in this process.) You can then take steps to

THE ALLERGENS

The most common allergen involved in hay fever is pollen – or, in fact, a protein on the surface of a grain of pollen. A hay fever sufferer may be allergic to any one – or several – of the huge number of different types or families of plants that produce pollen.

Other common allergens are mould spores, the droppings of the house dust mite, dried cat saliva and flakes of animal or insect skin or hair.

remove it from the child's environment. For example, keep windows closed on dry days during the season for the pollen to which your child is allergic, or vacuum the house often and thoroughly if the house dust mite is implicated.

The only long-term medical treatment for hay fever is desensitization, which involves a series of injections to teach the body to tolerate the allergen. They are not always effective, often have to be repeated yearly and can be dangerous.

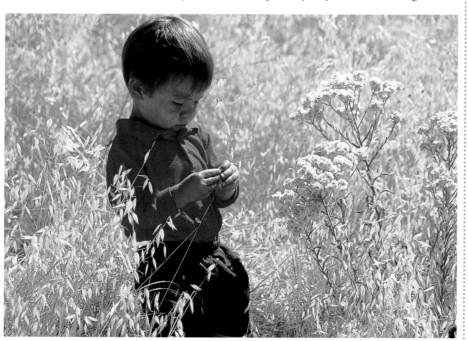

Enjoying nature
Because babies and toddlers have immature immune systems, they usually escape the unpleasantness of hay fever. However, some will develop the condition when they become older.

Coughs and colds

For an adult, having a cold may be uncomfortable, but it is far from serious. When a baby or child has a cold, however, there can sometimes – although rarely – be complications that require medical help.

A cold is an upper respiratory tract infection caused by a virus that is transmitted from one person to another by close contact – often by coughing or sneezing – and any of more than 100 different viruses may be responsible. Babies and children are particularly susceptible because their immune system does not develop fully until they reach the age of five.

Symptoms usually last for three to four days. They include a runny nose, sore throat, headache and mild fever, and there may also be coughing, sneezing, tiredness and minor aches and pains.

Treatment

Because a cold is a viral infection, antibiotics are not an effective treatment; however, they may be given to combat secondary bacterial infections. Instead, you should give your child plenty of fluids and encourage her to blow her nose when it becomes stuffy. You can ease any soreness around the nostrils by applying a thin layer of petroleum jelly.

Keep air in the room moist by placing wet towels or bowls of warm water over a radiator, and help your child breathe overnight by spraying a menthol preparation near her pillow (do not use it for babies, who should not use pillows; see pp.18–19). A high temperature can be reduced by giving your child children's paracetamol – never give a child less than 12 years old aspirin (see p.63).

Precautions

A cold is unlikely to give rise to any serious complications, but you should remember these points when a child or baby has one.

- During a severe cold, the virus can sometimes spread down to the lungs, causing either bronchitis or bronchiolitis (see opposite).
- A cold reduces the body's immune response, so a secondary bacterial infection of the ears, throat, sinuses or respiratory tract may develop.
- A cold can trigger an asthma attack in asthma sufferers (see pp.76–77).
- A baby with a blocked nose may find it difficult to feed; your doctor may suggest saline drops or a nasal decongestant.
- Call your doctor if a cold persists for more than 10 days or if your child's temperature continues to rise.

COUGHS

Coughing is a symptom of a cold, as well of other conditions such as bronchitis. A cough is a reflex action, caused by the stimulation of nerve endings in the throat, in which air is suddenly expelled to rid the nasal passages of excessive mucus or any foreign bodies.

A child often coughs when lying down because in this position any nasal discharge can drip down the back of her throat and stimulate the cough reflex.

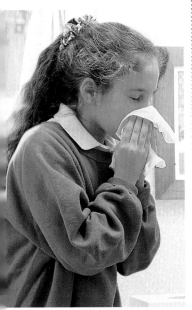

Keeping the passages clear
Encouraging your child to blow her nose will help prevent mucus from entering the lungs.

Bronchitis

The cause of bronchitis – which is an inflammation of the bronchi (the larger airways in the lungs) – may be viral or bacterial. Viral bronchitis occurs when the virus that causes a cold (opposite) or influenza spreads down the upper respiratory tract; bacterial bronchitis is usually an opportunistic, secondary infection that sets in when the immune system is weakened by another infection.

Symptoms may include a runny nose a few days prior to its onset, a persistent cough – it starts off dry, then produces phlegm – wheezing, shortness of breath and a slight fever. In viral bronchitis the phlegm is opaque; in bacterial bronchitis it is yellowish green. The problem usually clears up within three to four days, but bouts may recur during the winter until the immune system becomes mature.

You can give your child paracetamol – never aspirin – to reduce a fever. Do not give her a cough suppressant because it is important that the phlegm is coughed up. To encourage coughing, keep the air in her room moist and give her lots of fluids to loosen the phlegm. You can also lie your child over your knee and pat her back.

Consult your doctor if your child's temperature rises over 39°C (102.2°F), if the phlegm is coloured or if breathing is rapid. A diagnosis is made on the basis of the symptoms. The doctor may prescribe antibiotics if the infection is bacterial and, sometimes, a bronchodilator – a drug that widens the bronchioles.

SEE ALSO

Infectious diseases	**60–61**
Reye's syndrome and aspirin	**63**
Influenza	**65**
The lungs and respiration	**74–75**

Bronchiolitis

There is sometimes an epidemic of bronchiolitis during the late autumn and winter months. The cause of the condition may be any of the viruses that can cause a cold (opposite), but it results in inflammation of the tiny airways in the lungs – the bronchioles. Because they have such minuscule bronchioles, babies and toddlers are most severely affected, and the condition can, on occasion, prove fatal. Bronchiolitis can also trigger an asthma attack in asthma sufferers (see pp.76–77).

At the start of an attack, the symptoms are the same as those of a cold. These persist for two to three days, but then there may be wheezing and breathlessness, leading to rapid breathing with occasional long pauses. Low levels of oxygen in the blood may then lead to drowsiness and a reluctance to feed, and the lips may turn blue. An older infant may have only the symptoms of a cold or none at all.

Without complications, bronchiolitis clears up within 7 to 10 days and treatment at home is the same as for bronchitis. However, call a doctor immediately if there is any difficulty in breathing, drowsiness or the baby's lips turn blue. Support the child in an upright position to assist her breathing and oxygen uptake. The baby may have to be admitted to hospital to receive oxygen and intravenous food and fluids.

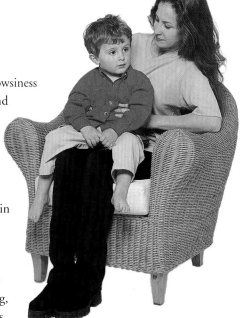

Sitting up

Holding a child snuggled against you in an upright position will help him breathe more easily.

Making steam

Steam can help relieve croup – a humidifier or bowls of steaming water add moisture to the air.

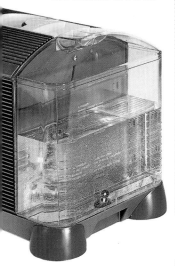

Croup

Laryngo-tracheo-bronchitis, commonly known as croup, is an infection of the larynx, trachea and bronchi. Usually, croup is caused by a viral infection of the larynx, which follows an upper respiratory tract infection, such as a cold, and spreads lower into the airway. Other, less common, causes of croup are a bacterial infection or a foreign body that has been inhaled.

Croup affects children between six months and four years old, and it normally occurs at night or in the early morning. In mild cases the symptoms are:
- Those of a cold for one or two days (when the cause of croup is a respiratory tract infection).
- A harsh barking cough – the croup – with a whistling sound when breathing in.
- A hoarse voice or cry.
- Some difficulty in breathing.

In such cases, care for the child in the same way as you would if he had a cold; recovery is normally within five days. However, you should always inform your doctor about an attack of croup; sometimes assessment by a specialist may be recommended.

In more severe cases, immediate medical attention may be necessary. Call your doctor at once if breathing becomes rapid or extremely difficult, or if the lips, tongue or body become grey or blue. While waiting for assistance, place the child in the bathroom and run the hot tap to moisturize the air quickly; hold him upright (but not in the water) to assist oxygen uptake. Hospital treatment may involve medicated inhalations and giving oxygen through a mask or, in extreme cases, through a tube passed into the lungs from the nose.

Epiglottitis

The epiglottis is a piece of cartilage by the base of the tongue; it prevents food from entering the trachea. In epiglottitis, which affects children between one and six years of age, the epiglottis becomes inflamed and swollen as a result of an infection by the *Haemophilus influenzae* bacterium. The condition is now rare, because the Hib vaccine against the bacterium is part of a baby's standard immunizations. However, if epiglottitis does occur, it can be severe and may stop air from reaching the lungs.

The onset of epiglottitis is sudden. Symptoms include a spasmodic cough and a sore throat; drooling because of the difficulty in swallowing; rasping breathing that quietens as the condition deteriorates; a high fever; and a bluish tinge to the lips and skin. Call for an ambulance straight away. Until help arrives, hold the child upright to help breathing and keep him calm – crying increases mucus production, which may further block the airway.

In hospital, antibiotics may be given intravenously and a tube may be passed into the larynx through the nose. In severe cases a hole may be cut in the trachea – a tracheotomy – below the site of the blockage. Recovery is usually complete within a week, and the child should become immune to the condition.

Tonsillitis and pharyngitis

Two conditions that affect the throat are tonsillitis and pharyngitis. They are often hard to differentiate because an infection of the tonsils usually also involves infection of the pharynx – the throat – and vice versa.

The tonsils are two almond-shaped masses of lymphatic tissue, which sit on either side of the entrance to the throat. They form a protective barrier against infections of the upper respiratory tract, in particular, the pharynx. Both the tonsils and the pharynx may become inflamed as a result of a viral infection, such as a cold, or a secondary bacterial infection, which is usually caused by streptococcal bacteria.

The two conditions are common in children, but their incidence decreases as children acquire immunity to common viruses. Symptoms include a sore throat, with pain and difficulty in swallowing, swollen neck glands and fever. In young children, there may also be abdominal pains and vomiting.

Home treatment is the same as for a cold, but call your doctor if the condition persists or the fever worsens 24 hours after its onset. You can give older children throat lozenges to suck, not chew.

Your doctor may prescribe antibiotics if a bacterial infection is suspected. A throat swab may be taken and cultured to confirm the diagnosis because there is a small risk that streptococcal bacteria can cause rheumatic fever. Although once common, surgical removal of the tonsils is now rarely considered – only when there are many episodes of infection and they don't appear to be getting less frequent.

The throat

Also called the pharynx, the throat can become sore and painful when infected. The tonsils and larynx are common sites of infection.

LARYNGITIS

Although laryngitis – an inflammation of the larynx – is usually caused by a viral infection, it can be caused by bacteria. The infection can spread to other parts of the airway and to the middle ear. Typical symptoms are a sore throat, fever, a dry cough and a cracked or hoarse voice. Sometimes the child temporarily loses his voice completely.

Until symptoms improve, give your child warm, soothing drinks. Increasing humidity in the room by placing damp towels or bowls of water on a hot radiator or by using a humidifier will also help. If breathing becomes noisy or difficult, consult your doctor right away – a swollen larynx can partially block the trachea.

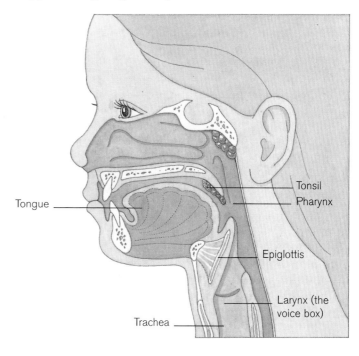

Tongue

Tonsil

Pharynx

Epiglottis

Larynx (the voice box)

Trachea

The ears and eyes

A child can learn about the environment around her by using her senses of hearing and sight. Sound waves and rays of light are translated by the ears and eyes, respectively, and sent to the brain for interpretation.

A baby who cannot hear will not be able to reproduce sounds, so her speech and language development will suffer. Poor eyesight will hamper a child in everything she does, and can even be dangerous – for example, she may not see a step and fall down it.

The ear

There are three parts to the ear: the outer ear, middle ear and inner ear. The pinna (the part of the ear that is visible) and the external auditory canal form the outer ear, which conveys sound waves to the middle ear, amplifying the sound as it does so. Sound vibrations land on the eardrum and are carried across the middle ear by

three tiny bones: the malleus, incus and stapes. Vibration of the stapes causes the fluid inside the spiral cochlea in the inner ear to vibrate. Hair cells in the organ of Corti inside the cochlea then transform the mechanical vibrations into electrical nerve impulses, which travel along the cochlear nerve to the brain for processing into the sounds that we perceive.

Babies should be able to hear from birth (indeed, it has been shown that the foetus is sensitive to sound), and it is essential to identify those children who have any impairment so that treatment can begin at once. There are two types of hearing impairment in children – conductive deafness, which affects

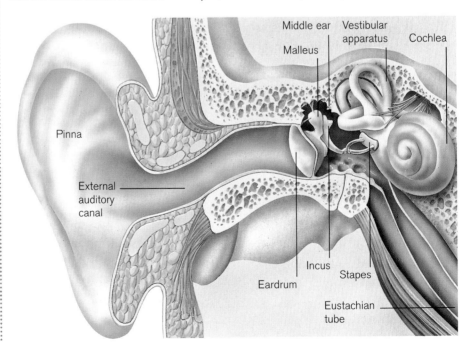

Anatomy of the ear

Sound entering the pinna passes along the external auditory canal to the middle ear and thence to the cochlea and the brain.

Middle ear   Vestibular apparatus   Cochlea

Malleus

Pinna

External auditory canal

Incus

Eardrum   Stapes

Eustachian tube

4 percent of children, and sensorineural deafness, which affects only 0.3 percent. Conductive deafness occurs when the sound waves are not conducted to the inner ear properly. This is often caused by glue ear (see pp.86–87).

Sensorineural deafness is caused by damage to the cochlear, or auditory, nerve. This may be genetic in origin – in about half of all cases – or it may occur because of intrauterine infection, severe jaundice or severe infection in childhood.

The eye

The pupil, lens and cornea at the front of the eye are only part of the optic pathway, which also includes the retina at the back of the eye. The shape of the lens can be altered to some extent by the ciliary muscles, which make it fatter to focus on near objects or thinner for far ones. This means the lens can refract, or bend, rays of light from an object so that they are in focus on the retina, with its light-sensitive rod and cone cells. The 120 million rods produce a coarse grey image; the 6 million cones provide detail and colour. These cells transmit messages through the optic nerve to the optic cortex, the part of the brain devoted to interpreting vision.

Newborn babies blink in response to a sudden bright light and turn toward a diffuse light at about a week. Any suspicion that your baby cannot see properly should be investigated at once.

One of the most common visual problems in children occurs when the lens is unable to focus the incoming rays of light on to the retina. In myopia, or short-sightedness, rays of light from close objects focus correctly, but light from distant objects focuses in front of the retina; this is because the shape of the eye is too long or the converging powers of the cornea and lens are not great enough.

The problem is solved by placing a diverging, or concave, lens in front of the eye. In hypermetropia, or long-sightedness, the rays of light from distant objects focus on the retina, but light from a close object is brought into focus behind the retina – the shape of the eye is too short or the focusing power of the cornea and lens is insufficient. This can be overcome by placing a convex, or converging, lens in front of the eye. Astigmatism occurs when the cornea is not curved evenly, causing

SEE ALSO

Ear problems	86–87
Eye problems	88–89
Hearing difficulties	202–203
Visual problems	204–205

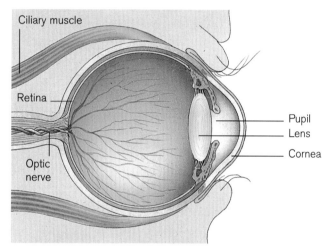

Anatomy of the eye

Light from an object enters the eye through the cornea and is brought into focus – but inverted – on the retina. The image is then sent by the optic nerve to the brain.

an uneven focus in different planes; it is corrected with a specially shaped lens.

There are other eye problems such as a squint (see pp.204–205) and, rarely, retinal detachment and cataracts (when the lens becomes cloudy or opaque). One in every 20 babies is colour blind; it is rare in girls and only becomes a problem when certain jobs must be excluded. In the most common type red and green are indistinguishable. Premature babies are susceptible to certain eye problems, so they will be examined before leaving hospital.

Ear problems

There are several causes of pain in the ear in children. The most common of these is acute otitis media, which can sometimes lead to glue ear. Most cases get better without treatment and only need monitoring by a doctor.

Earache is common in children, and parents may be faced with a very distressed child screaming with pain in the early hours of the morning. While older children are able to say which ear hurts, babies and young children tend to pull at the affected ear and may be quite unwell with fever and even vomiting.

Otitis media

Ear examination

If the doctor suspects that your child has otitis media, he will examine his ear with an otoscope. In the early stages the eardrum will appear red and withdrawn, but later on it will bulge outward.

The middle ear may be infected by a virus (usually the adenovirus) or by bacteria. The pain occurs when the Eustachian tube becomes inflamed and swells, leading to a build-up of fluid in the middle ear, which presses on the eardrum (the fluid normally drains down the tube). If the cause is bacteria, there may also be pus. The child usually has an upper respiratory tract infection several days before and may only complain of pain. More often, he is hot, miserable, unwell and doesn't want to eat.

The infection usually disappears after a few days, and in children who are well apart from earache, the only treatment needed is decongestant nose drops to reduce swelling and paracetamol for pain. Local heat applied by placing a well-wrapped, warm hot water bottle under the affected ear can soothe pain. Never drip warm oil into the ear. Antibiotics are often prescribed, but they often make little difference in relieving the symptoms.

Sometimes the eardrum ruptures, releasing the fluid and pus and relieving the pain. It can be distressing for both parents and child to find blood and pus in the outer ear or on the pillow, but the eardrum usually heals within a few weeks, as long as the ear is kept dry and no further infection occurs. Even so, it is advisable to take the child to the doctor after an eardrum has burst.

In some children the fluid in the middle ear persists and the chronic condition called glue ear results. It is important, therefore, that children with otitis media are examined a couple of weeks after the initial attack to check that the eardrum and hearing have returned to normal.

Glue ear

The largest cause of fluctuating or variable deafness in childhood is glue ear, the common name for what is now known

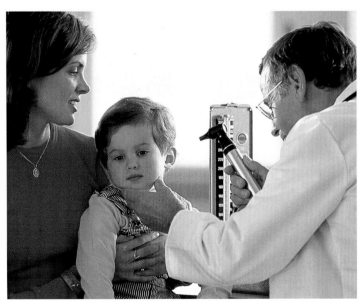

as chronic otitis media with effusion. A sticky mucuslike fluid, which is produced by the lining of the middle ear, becomes trapped because it is unable to drain away down the Eustachian tube. The tube may be inflamed, or it may be blocked at its lower end by enlarged adenoids.

Glue ear is more common in boys and in children with a cleft palate. One-third of children under the age of six are affected at some stage, but most do not require treatment and need only to be monitored.

The main symptom is impairment of hearing. The loss of hearing is variable and is worse in winter. Parents and teachers need to speak clearly to the child and should make sure that he hears what has been said. Making sure the child faces the speaker will help him to hear better.

In most children, the problem resolves of its own accord as they get older and the Eustachian tube grows longer and wider. Hearing should be monitored regularly. If the child has large adenoids blocking the end of the Eustachian tube, they may need to be removed surgically to allow the fluid from the middle ear to drain away freely. Grommets may be inserted if the fluid persists (see box, right).

Other causes of earache

Inflammation or blockage of the Eustachian tube hinders the free drainage of fluid from the middle ear. Pain may be felt in the ear when all the air in the middle ear is forced out and a negative pressure is formed. The condition can be treated to a degree by inhaling steam and taking decongestants.

Pain from tonsillitis or dental infection may be felt as earache because of the shared nerve supply. Rarely, a boil in the external ear canal or a foreign body in the canal may cause pain; these will be seen easily on examining the affected ear.

Otitis externa, inflammation of the external ear canal, can be caused by a bacterial infection, seborrhoeic dermatitis or atopic eczema (see pp.102–103). There may be a discharge from the canal, with pain and itching. Treatment is with anti-inflammatory ear drops and antibiotics.

How to give ear drops

The child should lie down on a bed or across your lap, with the affected ear uppermost. A pillow under his head will help to keep it steady and comfortable.

When using a dropper, it should be held just above the canal entrance, and the drops deposited gently in the ear. Many drops now come in plastic bottles with pointed nozzles; the bottle should be inverted and squeezed gently until the correct number of drops has been given.

SEE ALSO

Routine health contacts	**30–31**
Tonsillitis and pharyngitis	**83**
The ears and eyes	**84–85**
Hearing difficulties	**202–203**

GROMMETS FOR GLUE EAR

If hearing fails to improve in a child suffering from glue ear, a grommet (below, right) may need to be inserted. This is a tiny plastic tube that is placed through the eardrum. It allows air to enter the middle ear, which, in turn, displaces the fluid down the Eustachian tube. Fluid should not discharge back through the grommet into the outer ear unless further infection occurs.

Some specialists recommend that children with grommets should not swim at all and should wear ear plugs at bathtime and hair washing time. Others allow swimming, provided that the child does not dive or swim underwater.

A grommet usually stays in place for about nine months, after which time it will be extruded naturally and may be found in the ear canal or on the pillow in the morning. The hole in the eardrum heals over by itself, although it may leave a little scar. Occasionally the glue ear returns and another grommet is necessary.

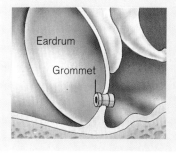

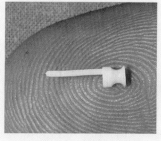

Eye problems

The most common eye problems in children respond to simple treatment. However, because they tend to be infectious, scrupulous hygiene must be observed to avoid spreading them to other family members.

Conjunctivitis is the eye problem that most often affects children. Antibiotic eye drops or ointment are prescribed when the conjunctivitis is thought to be bacterial in origin; anti-allergy eye drops may need to be used regularly during the hay fever season.

Giving eye drops or ointment to babies and children is never easy. Let your child know that it won't be painful and instruct her to sit or lie with her head tilted backward, looking up at the ceiling. When placing drops or ointment into the eye, the nozzle of the bottle or tube should be close to the eye but should not touch it. If both eyes are affected, two

Giving eye drops
While gently holding down the lower lid, place the drops in the trough between the lid and the eye – do not touch the eye. Only use eye drops prescribed by the doctor, not proprietary eye drops or eye baths.

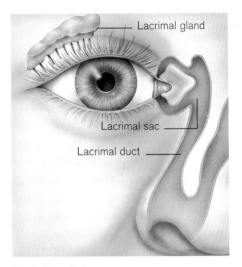

Blocked tear duct
The lacrimal gland secretes tears, which drain through a duct into the nose. Sometimes it is blocked in newborns, but it does not need treatment unless the condition persists.

bottles or tubes may be prescribed so that one can be used for each eye. Drops should not be dripped from a height on to the front of the eye – this causes the child to blink, so the drop hits the closed eyelid and runs down the cheek.

Blocked tear duct

Occasionally, the tear, or nasolacrimal, duct does not open properly in a newborn, so her tears are unable to drain away and the baby has a perpetually watery, sticky eye. This generally looks far more serious than it is. In the majority of cases, the condition corrects itself as the baby grows older. Parents are taught how

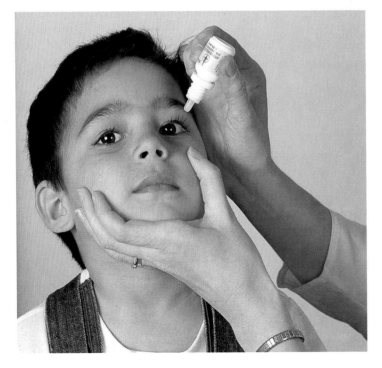

to keep the eye clean, and they may be taught how to massage the lacrimal sac at the inner part of the eyelid, by the bridge of the nose, to encourage the tear duct to open. Antibiotic drops or ointment are needed only if there is an infection.

If the problem persists after the first year of life, the tear duct will be gently explored by an ophthalmic surgeon while the baby is under general anaesthesia. The duct should not be syringed or probed by anyone else.

SEE ALSO

Your newborn baby	**10–11**
Routine health contacts	**30–31**
Allergies and hay fever	**78–79**
The ears and eyes	**84–85**

EYE INFECTIONS AND INFLAMMATIONS

Problem	Cause and symptoms	Treatment
Conjunctivitis 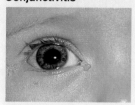	This condition occurs when the conjunctiva, the outermost layer of the eye, which also lines the eyelids, becomes inflamed. The inflammation may be caused by a bacterial or viral infection or by an allergy. Chemical conjunctivitis may occur if an irritating substance splashes into the eye. The eye itself appears red and feels sore and possibly gritty; the eyelids may be puffy. There is no visual disturbance, although looking at a bright light may be uncomfortable. A thick, greenish yellow discharge is common with bacterial conjunctivitis. This sometimes causes the eyelids to stick together and can be distressing for a child who is unable to open her eyes on waking.	The doctor may prescribe antibiotic drops or ointment. Clean the affected eye gently, using clean cotton wool balls soaked in cool, boiled tap water. (Boil the cotton wool in the water and let them cool. Cover the pan and keep it in the refrigerator; lift the cotton wool out with a clean spoon.) If the doctor suggests adding salt to the water, it should taste no saltier than tears. Using a separate ball for each eye, swab the eye gently from the corner nearest the nose outward. Wash your hands thoroughly before and after the procedure because conjunctivitis is contagious. To stop it from spreading, the child should use a separate face flannel and towel kept apart from the rest of the family's.
Blepharitis	Associated with seborrhoeic dermatitis or caused by a bacterial infection, blepharitis is an inflammation of the eyelids with redness and scaling where the lashes enter the lid. The eyelids are itchy and sore; there may be a build-up of scales that is hard to remove.	Using clean cotton wool balls (see above), clean the eyelids carefully twice a day to remove the scales and any greasy debris. If there is an infection, antibiotic ointment can be massaged into the edge of the lid several times a day.
Sty (hordeolum) 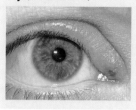	A sty is a tender, painful lump in the upper or lower eyelid, which is usually caused by a staphylococcal infection. It forms an abscess around the base of an eyelash and sometimes looks like a spot or pimple that is about to burst.	The sty often bursts spontaneously, discharging the pus it contains and relieving the pain. Local heat applied with a clean, hot flannel or cotton wool ball (see above) may help to relieve the pain. A prescribed antibiotic ointment may be massaged into the affected area, but there is no real evidence that this treatment is effective.
Meibomian cyst (chalazion)	This is a firm, uncomfortable swelling of the eyelid caused by blockage of the duct of 1 of the about 30 meibomian glands in each eyelid. The glands secrete an oily substance that lubricates the eyelids and contributes to the tear film on the eye's surface. The lump may press on the surface of the eye, causing some blurring of vision.	A meibomian cyst usually gets better or goes away without treatment, but if it persists, it may need to be scraped away under general or local anaesthesia.

Digestion

The digestive system is essentially an extremely long tube that starts at the mouth and finishes at the rectum. Parts of this tube, along with associated organs, have evolved to carry out particular functions.

As food passes through the tube, it is mixed with digestive juices that break down complex molecules to simpler forms, which are then absorbed by the body to produce the energy needed for all its functions. The unabsorbed residue is eliminated at the end of the tube.

Digestion begins as soon as food is placed in the mouth. The salivary glands secrete saliva into the mouth to lubricate the food and make swallowing easier. Ptyalin, an enzyme in saliva, begins to break down the starch. The mastication, or chewing, of food breaks it down into smaller pieces, which assists swallowing and produces a larger area on which the enzyme can act.

Swallowing itself is a complex process that involves the mouth, pharynx and upper part of the oesophagus. The swallowed bolus of food travels down the oesophagus into the stomach, where it is mixed with a variety of chemicals, known as gastric juice, ground up and digested further.

The intestines

The next part of the digestive tract is the intestines, or bowel. The small intestine starts with a short section, the duodenum, followed by a much longer jejunum and an even longer ileum. The duodenum is the main site of lipolysis, or fat digestion, in adults; however, in newborn babies lipolysis occurs in the stomach. It is in the jejunum and ileum that most of the nutrients in food are absorbed into the blood, which carries them to the liver for further digestion.

Continuing from the small intestine is the large intestine, which is made up of the colon and the appendix. No nutrients are absorbed in the colon, but it reabsorbs water so the material it contains becomes more solid as it moves toward the final part of the digestive tract.

The digestive system

Food passes from the mouth to the stomach, where secretions (see box, opposite) assist in digestion. Nutrients and water are absorbed in the intestines before waste is expelled from the rectum.

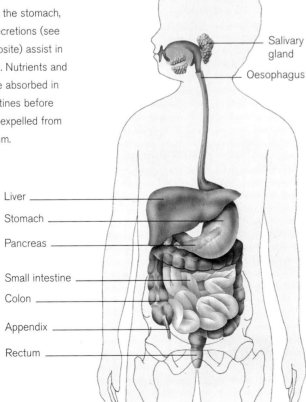

Salivary gland

Oesophagus

Liver

Stomach

Pancreas

Small intestine

Colon

Appendix

Rectum

The last part of the digestive tract is the rectum, from which the semi-solid waste material is finally eliminated in the form of faeces.

The liver and pancreas

Although not part of the digestive tube, the liver and pancreas play an important role in digestion. The pancreas secretes a large quantity of fluid rich in enzymes that assist in digesting food. The liver secretes bile – which helps break down fats so that they can be absorbed in the small intestine – makes cholesterol and plays a vital part in protein metabolism. It also stores glucose as glycogen and can call on this store when the blood sugar level falls (see pp.137–139).

What can go wrong

Problems can arise in any part of the digestive tract. Sometimes a part is not properly formed or connected during embryological development, leading to a congenital abnormality – a problem that is present from birth. With oesophageal atresia, for example, the oesophagus is not formed properly, so the baby is unable to swallow and chokes on the first feed. At the lower end of the tract there may be an imperforate anus, a condition in which the baby cannot pass any motions.

The small intestine in a baby or child may become obstructed for any one of a number of reasons. Sometimes it twists around on itself in a volvulus (see box, p.92); in a baby, the blockage may be due to impacted meconium – the first faeces passed by a newborn baby (see pp.12–13). In the large intestine, the most common cause of obstruction is Hirschsprung's disease. The typical symptoms of this disorder are vomiting, abdominal pain and unusual delay in passing the first motion.

Appendicitis, an acute inflammation of the appendix, is a common cause of abdominal pain and vomiting in children. Infections of the gastrointestinal tract can cause gastroenteritis, with profuse diarrhoea, vomiting and the danger of dehydration if the appropriate fluid intake cannot be maintained. In rarer cases, a chronic inflammatory bowel disorder may lead to poor weight gain and the passage of blood and mucus in the motions.

Some medical conditions lead to malabsorption of food, with consequently poor weight gain and failure to thrive. In cystic fibrosis (see p.148), for example, because the pancreas does not function properly, fat is not absorbed well, so foul-smelling, fatty stools are passed. In coeliac disease (see pp.98–99), sensitivity to the gluten in wheat and rye causes structural changes in the jejunum, which affect the normal process of digestion and lead to malabsorption. The child may suffer from vomiting and diarrhoea, abdominal distension, anaemia and muscle wasting – all of which can be reversed if gluten is excluded from the diet.

Infestations with parasites (see p.97) are a cause of malabsorption and poor health in the developing world, in particular; however, they also occur in people living in industrialized countries.

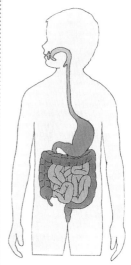

Going through the system
After 1 minute in the mouth and 10 seconds in the oesophagus, food stays 2–4 hours in the stomach, 1–6 hours in the small intestine and 10 hours to a few days in the large intestine.

HOW THE STOMACH FUNCTIONS

The cells of the stomach produce various substances, including pepsinogen – a protein-digesting enzyme – and intrinsic factor, which is essential for the absorption of vitamin B_{12}. Gastrin is a hormone that causes the secretion of hydrochloric acid, which is important for protein digestion and also acts to reduce the number of microorganisms living in the stomach.

With all the acid and digestive enzymes it contains, it is amazing that the stomach does not digest itself. However, mucus is secreted by the cells lining the stomach and bicarbonate is also produced to act as a buffer against the hydrochloric acid. When this mechanism fails, the stomach wall is damaged and an ulcer is formed.

Abdominal pain

All children experience abdominal pain at some stage. Babies and infants tend to pull their knees up to their chest, leaving parents in little doubt that they are in discomfort. Older children can describe the pain.

Signs of distress

Crying and knees drawn up to the chest are the classic symptoms of colic in a baby.

There are many manifestations and causes of abdominal pain – it may come on suddenly or be recurrent and it may be accompanied by other symptoms such as fever, diarrhoea or vomiting. The pain may be constant or intermittent and can be a dull ache or a sharp pain. Some conditions, such as colic, are more common in babies, while others, such as appendicitis, occur mostly in children over five years of age. No specific cause will be found for abdominal pain in almost half of children over two years old. This is labelled acute nonspecific abdominal pain or recurrent abdominal pain if it is a regular occurrence.

The appendix is a small wormlike protrusion of the large intestine. It may become inflamed, causing acute appendicitis, and if left untreated, it may burst, leading to peritonitis or an abscess. It accounts for about one-third of all cases of acute abdominal pain in children admitted to hospital.

Colic is an extremely common problem in young babies, however, it is not known what causes it. Babies with colic seem to produce a lot of wind and this may come from the fermentation of lactose, contained in milk. Another possible cause is thought to be intestinal spasm.

Intussusception is a rare condition affecting babies between 3 and 18 months of age, in which a portion of the bowel telescopes in on itself. The affected piece of bowel becomes swollen, its blood supply may be jeopardized and the intestine may become obstructed.

Mesenteric adenitis, in which some lymph nodes in the abdomen become inflamed, is a cause of acute abdominal pain in children. It can be difficult to

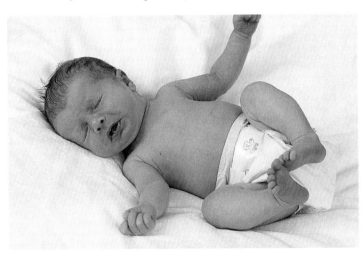

RECURRENT ABDOMINAL PAIN

Some children suffer from recurrent abdominal pain, which often appears to have no cause. This syndrome may affect a child between the ages of 2 and 13, but it usually begins after the age of 5. About 10 percent of schoolchildren have recurrent abdominal pain. The pain tends to be felt in the centre of the abdomen, and many children vomit. In some children, there is also diarrhoea, while others suffer from headaches between attacks. This condition is thought to be associated with stress and anxiety, both at school and at home (see pp.186–187). The child may be bullied at school or find learning difficult. At home, there may be arguments or other pressure.

One rare physical cause is recurrent volvulus, in which a loop of small intestine twists around on itself, obstructing the bowel. If the child starts to lose weight, has an unexplained temperature or starts to pass blood or mucus in the stools, she should see a doctor.

distinguish between mesenteric adenitis and acute appendicitis, but there are several distinguishing features.

Meckel's diverticulum is a type of protrusion of the terminal ileum, a part of the small intestine. It may become acutely inflamed causing severe lower abdominal pain on the left side. It can also become twisted – causing a volvulus – or cause an intussusception. It may contain some gastric tissue that can ulcerate and bleed, leading to blood in the motions.

SEE ALSO

Helping your child
in hospital   56–57

Food allergies and
intolerances   98–99

TYPES OF ABDOMINAL PAIN

Condition	Symptoms	Treatment
Appendicitis	Your child may feel pain in the bottom right-hand corner of the abdomen to begin with. She won't eat, has a slight temperature and usually vomits. There is tenderness in the area of the appendix, and she may cry if it is pressed. The pain may increase if the pressure is removed suddenly. It is better to ask her to puff out her stomach as much as she can, then to draw it in as thin as she can and watch her face for signs of pain.	The appendix should be removed before it bursts and its contents contaminate the abdomen, possibly causing peritonitis. It can be removed by an appendicectomy, using a small opening that requires only a few stitches or clips to close it up. The child will need to stay in hospital for a couple of days and will have to take a week or so off school. She will not be able to participate in sports for several weeks.
Colic	Colic affects both bottle- and breastfed babies. The baby is otherwise healthy and well but suffers from bouts of apparent abdominal pain, usually in the evenings. The knees are drawn up to the chest, the baby cries constantly and the only relief seems to come from being walked around in an upright position for hours on end.	The drugs that are prescribed may or may not be useful. In severe cases, a bottlefed baby may be fed a lactose-free formula and a breastfeeding mother may have to exclude cow's milk from her diet. A change of diet should only be on advice from the doctor or health visitor. Colic usually clears up by the end of the third or fourth month.
Intussusception	The baby may vomit and have bouts of screaming and drawing the knees up to her chest. She looks pale, although screaming babies usually turn red in the face. In between attacks, the baby may seem her usual self or be very quiet. The stools are normal in the early stages, but later bloodstained mucus is passed in the nappy.	To confirm the diagnosis, an abdominal X-ray or ultrasound examination may be needed. Immediate surgery is required if the baby is severely ill. In less serious cases, a special X-ray technique can straighten the bowel by using pressure. Some children need surgery to correct or remove the affected part of the bowel.
Mesenteric adenitis	The child may have symptoms of an upper respiratory tract infection with a headache, enlarged neck glands, inflamed lymph nodes and a temperature above 38°C (100°F). The child does not usually vomit. The abdominal pain is not severe and is felt in the centre of the abdomen.	There is no treatment for mesenteric adenitis; the pain goes away as the lymph nodes become less inflamed.
Meckel's diverticulum	This is a rare cause of acute abdominal pain. Symptoms are similar to those of acute appendicitis (see above), except the pain is felt in the left lower corner of the abdomen rather than the right.	A special scan may be used to make a diagnosis. If confirmed, surgery to remove the protrusion, similar to an appendicectomy (see above), is necessary.

Pyloric stenosis, reflux and common hernias

Posseting, when a baby brings up some of his feed, is normal, but if all or a large part of his feed is always brought up, the cause may be a serious disorder.

In pyloric stenosis, the pyloric muscle at the lower end of the stomach becomes thickened, so food cannot pass through it easily and the baby vomits up the whole feed shortly after feeding. The vomiting is forceful and may travel more than a metre (3 ft) – this is known as projectile vomiting. Boys are affected five times more often than girls, and first-born children more often than others.

The trouble usually starts at about three weeks old, with occasional vomiting after a feed, but soon progresses so that the baby vomits violently after every feed. The vomit may contain some blood but is not stained green with bile.

The baby will not appear to look concerned and will have a good appetite.

Constipation is common, although loose, greenish motions may be passed. Sometimes it is possible to see peristalsis (involuntary contractions) through the abdominal wall and to feel the thickened pylorus in the abdomen while the baby is feeding. If the condition is left untreated, the baby will become dehydrated and lose weight.

The stenosis is rectified by Ramstedt's operation – a simple procedure in which an incision is made in the thickened pyloric muscle while the baby is under general anaesthesia. It is usually successful, and the baby will feed normally a few hours afterward.

Gastro-oesophageal reflux and hiatus hernia

One common cause of vomiting is gastro-oesophageal reflux (GOR), which is more likely to occur in premature and bottlefed babies. In this condition, the valve between the oesophagus and stomach does not function properly and allows the stomach contents to flow back into the oesophagus.

Shortly after each feed the baby will vomit copiously. He may be obviously distressed, cry a good deal and arch his back during feeding. The lower end of the oesophagus may become inflamed as a result of contact with the acidic stomach contents. Sometimes the area bleeds, and the vomit may contain a little blood. The

Pyloric stenosis

This condition occurs when the pyloric muscle in the lower stomach is so thick that food cannot pass easily into the duodenum, which leads to the intestines.

Stomach

Duodenum

Pyloric muscle

baby must be observed while feeding and examined carefully to exclude other causes of vomiting. In most cases, the diagnosis can be made after examination. In some cases, special X-rays and a study of the level of acidity at the bottom of the oesophagus confirm the diagnosis. In rare cases, the doctor may use a gastroscope to look inside the oesophagus and stomach and take a fragment of tissue to assess the level of inflammation.

Several treatments are available, which are used separately or in combination. The first step is to feed the baby in an upright position and to keep him in this position for some time after the feed. The feed may need to be thickened with a special powder. Drugs that form a layer on top of the feed and help to keep it down may be prescribed, as may special preparations to cut down the amount of acid produced by the stomach, thereby relieving the oesophagitis. Normally, the reflux improves as the baby gets older.

There may also be a hiatus hernia, in which the upper part of the stomach projects through the opening in the diaphragm; some cases may need surgery.

Strangulated inguinal hernia

A hernia is formed when a piece of bowel, or intestine, protrudes through an opening in the abdominal wall. In a child, an inguinal hernia is due to the late closure, or failure to close, of part of the inguinal canal through which the testis descends. This may explain why it is more common in boys and why it may be associated with an undescended testicle (see pp.160–161).

It is seen as a swelling in the groin, which may come and go. Sometimes a piece of bowel becomes trapped inside the hernia, forming a strangulated hernia, which may cause severe lower abdominal pain and vomiting. The blood supply

to the trapped bowel is cut off and permanent damage may result unless the baby is operated on as soon as possible.

Umbilical hernia

Some babies are born with a protruding navel, or umbilical hernia, in which the intestine pushes through at the navel, where the abdominal wall may be weak. It is not related to the way in which the umbilical cord was clamped, nor is it formed because the baby's abdomen was not bound after birth. An umbilical hernia is more common in Afro-Caribbean babies and does not usually cause any problems. The hernia tends to become smaller as the baby grows, but if it doesn't disappear, it may need repairing.

SEE ALSO

Bottlefeeding	33
Abdominal pain	92–93
Vomiting, diarrhoea and constipation	96–97

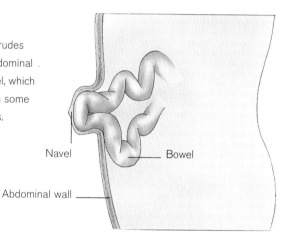

Umbilical hernia

The bowel protrudes through the abdominal wall at the navel, which may be weak in some newborn babies.

Navel

Bowel

Abdominal wall

HIRSCHSPRUNG'S DISEASE

This is a rare cause of constipation in newborns, occurring in 1 in 4,500 births. Typically, the baby does not pass the first meconium stool within the first 24 hours of life (see pp.12–13). The constipation continues, the abdomen enlarges, the baby refuses to feed, then begins to bring up bile-stained vomit. The problem is due to the absence of the normal nerve supply to a part of the large bowel, which remains contracted and immobile – much like a lead pipe – when it should be distending and moving with peristalsis.

Once suspected, the diagnosis is confirmed by a barium enema X-ray and a biopsy of the rectum. Surgery is then necessary to remove the affected segment and join the healthy sections.

Vomiting, diarrhoea and constipation

Almost every child will experience a bout of vomiting, diarrhoea or constipation. These are often minor symptoms, and they can usually be cared for at home.

Babies often bring up part of their feed. This is called posseting and is not a serious problem. As long as the baby gains weight, there is no cause for concern.

An older child's vomiting may be intermittent or continuous and sometimes the vomit contains blood or bile. The child may complain of abdominal pain or a headache and may be feverish (see pp.54–55) and dehydrated. Among the conditions that can cause vomiting are tonsillitis (see p.83), migraine (see p.166), meningitis (see pp.66–67), pertussis (see p.70), reflux, hernias and abdominal disorders. Vomiting is also a symptom of poisoning (see p.217). A common cause of vomiting and nausea is travel, or motion, sickness, which can be treated with anti-sick pills.

Treatment begins by finding out the cause of the vomiting and correcting it. Fluids have to be replaced either by mouth or, in severe cases, by a tube passed through the nose into the stomach or by intravenous drip.

Diarrhoea and vomiting

Gastroenteritis is the most common cause of diarrhoea and vomiting. About half of the cases in children under five years old are caused by viruses. Vomiting often precedes diarrhoea by a few hours and there may be abdominal pain. Younger children and babies become dehydrated more rapidly than older ones, particularly if they are unable to keep down any fluids taken by mouth. Oral rehydration therapy is the mainstay of treatment (opposite).

Otitis media (see p.86), chest infections, urinary tract infections, appendicitis, pyloric stenosis and intussusception can

FOOD POISONING

Cause	Symptoms
Salmonella Raw meat, poultry, sausages and eggs	Diarrhoea and vomiting 12 to 36 hours after infection; the attack may be brief, but the bacteria can be present in the motions for a prolonged period.
Escherichia coli (E. coli) Contaminated food or water	There are five different syndromes – all have diarrhoea of varying severity, some with renal failure.
Campylobacter Unpasteurized milk and raw poultry	Vomiting, abdominal pain, diarrhoea with blood, and fever. Symptoms start up to a week after infection.
Shigella A type of dysentery in contaminated water and food	Abdominal pain, vomiting, watery diarrhoea, aches, fever, followed by stools with mucus and blood. Symptoms begin one to seven days after infection and last about a week.
Listeria Soft cheeses, shellfish, fish, precooked foods, salads, pâtés, undercooked poultry	Fever, conjunctivitis, swollen glands and a rash. They appear six weeks after infection and it can take months to recover completely.
Clostridium perfingens Contaminated meat	Severe vomiting; starts 12 to 24 hours after infection and is short-lived.
Bacillus cereus Contaminated rice	Severe vomiting; begins 2 to 12 hours after infection and is short-lived.

WORMS

Infestations of threadworms may occur in some children. They can be identified as short, white threads in the stools or can be see around the anus at night when the child is sleeping. They may cause considerable anal and vulval itching and can cause abdominal pain. The worms can be eradicated by a single dose of a drug taken by mouth. The whole family should be treated and a second dose of treatment given a few weeks later if the worms persist.

Infestations with other worms – roundworm, hookworm or tapeworm – are much less common in industrialized countries. Specific drugs are available to treat each infestation.

all cause diarrhoea and vomiting in children. Food intolerance may cause diarrhoea in babies. Inflammatory bowel disorders, which are rare in children, may cause diarrhoea, often with blood and mucus in the stools.

If diarrhoea is protracted, a specimen may be sent to a laboratory to identify the organism causing the symptoms. Some bacteria are treated with antibiotics, but this is the exception rather than the rule.

Oral rehydration therapy

Special solutions that combine sugar and mineral salts enhance fluid absorption in the gut. You should give a child with severe vomiting or diarrhoea small amounts of rehydration fluid at room temperature every 15 to 30 minutes.

Do not stop breastfeeding a baby. Give the rehydration fluid, mixed with cooled boiled water, by spoon. You can give bland solids to older children, but they may not want to eat much. Parents used to be advised to give only clear fluids, but this is no longer thought to be necessary.

Severe dehydration and the inability to take any fluid by mouth will mean hospitalizing a baby to give her fluids through a nasogastric tube or into a vein.

Constipation

The frequency of passing stools is not important, providing they are normal and soft and their passage causes no discomfort. Constipation occurs when there is pain and difficulty in passing stools, and they emerge as hard, dry lumps. Pain in passing stools can cause a child to withhold them, which can lead to the formation of a distended rectum that can hold even more stools. Eventually, there is faecal overflow and soiling.

A child who is constipated should be seen by a doctor. The child's diet will be assessed to see whether it contains enough fluids and fibre. Drugs that soften the faeces may help the child pass normal stools without discomfort. Other drugs speed the passage of the stool.

A small tear, or fissure, at the edge of the anus may cause pain. Any local anal soreness can be treated so that defecation is not painful. Sometimes, constipation may be an indication of a blockage such as in Hirschsprung's disease (see p.95).

SEE ALSO
Digestion   **90–91**
Abdominal pain   **92–93**
Pyloric stenosis, reflux
and common hernias   **94–95**

Baby's first food

When weaning a baby on to her first solid foods, avoid foods that contain sugar. They can cause diarrhoea in some babies – and sugar contributes to tooth decay.

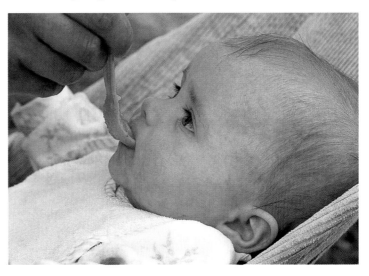

Food allergies and intolerances

A food allergy occurs when the body's defence system responds abnormally to a food; an intolerance occurs when the enzyme to digest a protein in a food is missing.

Increasing numbers of children are allergic to peanuts – one of the most common foods to trigger an allergic response – possibly because of early exposure to peanut protein in the womb or in breast milk if their mother eats peanuts. Other foods that can trigger an allergic response, in which the body's defence system attacks an otherwise innocuous substance, include milk and other dairy products; eggs; fish and shellfish; wheat and wheat products; other nuts; citrus fruit, melons and fruit with seeds (such as strawberries); and chocolate. (In some people, oil on the peel of citrus fruit may trigger the response; the fruit can be eaten if someone else first removes the peel.)

The allergic reaction may be fairly mild and hardly noticed at all, for example, there may be a mild rash that goes away in a few hours. However, there may be a very severe reaction in some children, with swelling of the mouth and throat that leads to difficulty in swallowing and breathing and eventual collapse. The child should be taken to an accident and emergency department immediately if he starts to develop swelling of the face or has any difficulty breathing. If your child is severely allergic to peanuts, it may be recommended that he carries a syringe filled with adrenaline with him at all times.

Pregnant women with a strong family history of allergic responses to certain

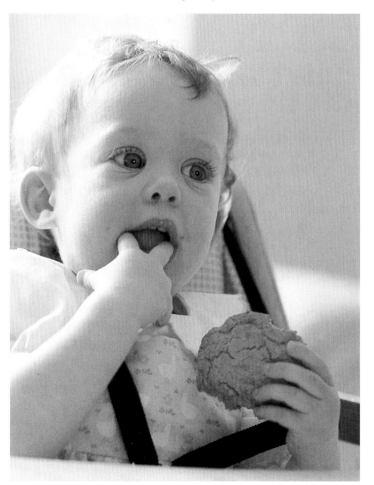

Gluten-free rusk

If your teething baby has coeliac disease, you can buy her special gluten-free rusks, which are available on prescription. Other foods that have been formulated without gluten, such as bread and biscuits, are also available.

foods are best advised to avoid those foods during pregnancy and while breastfeeding. Whole peanuts should not be given to any child under the age of five years and foods containing peanuts should not be given to children under the age of three who are likely to be sensitive to them. It may take only a trace of the protein to bring on a severe reaction. For other foods to avoid when weaning your child from breast milk or formula, see page 35.

Coeliac disease

In coeliac disease, the digestive tract cannot digest the gluten in wheat and rye. It is thought to be due to the lack of an enzyme in the wall of the intestine that prevents the breakdown of gliaden, part of gluten. The problem becomes apparent when cereals are introduced into the baby's diet after four months of age. The baby is miserable, irritable and has no appetite. There is a general failure to thrive and put on weight. Bulky, pale, offensive stools are passed because of the poor absorption of fat. The baby may vomit, lose weight and have a distended abdomen. There may also be iron deficiency anaemia.

KNOWING THE INGREDIENTS

Some foods may have to be eliminated from a child's diet altogether. It is important to read all food labels. If you have a young child, make sure you alert the parents of any friends he visits, as well as his nursery or primary school.

When eating in restaurants, inquire about the ingredients in the items on the menu. If the waiter or chef cannot guarantee that they can serve a dish without the problematic ingredient, ask them to prepare simple, plain items such as poached meat without a sauce and steamed vegetables.

Once coeliac diesase is suspected, the diagnosis can be made by taking a biopsy from the small intestine to examine the cells that line it. Blood tests may also show specific antibodies against gliaden.

All gluten must be totally excluded from the diet. This means getting special gluten-free breads and biscuits on prescription. If the child is deficient in iron, folic acid or other nutrients, he may need supplements. An immediate improvement will be noticed, with an increase in weight and in the child's general wellbeing. A gluten-free diet will need to be followed for life in all but a few cases.

Food intolerances

Coelic disease is one type of food intolerance, and there are others – but they are not as common as some parents assume. Babies and young children often have colic and diarrhoea, but this does not mean that they are reacting to cow's milk. However, after a bout of gastroenteritis (see pp.96–97), babies under the age of six months may become temporarily intolerant of the milk sugar lactose. This problem is due to a short-term shortage of lactase, the enzyme that metabolizes lactose.

Some children cannot digest lactose in cow's milk at all because they don't make enough lactase. The symptoms are wind, diarrhoea and abdominal cramps and, in the long term, failure to thrive and put on weight. Such children can be given yogurt, in which the lactose has already been converted, and some can tolerate hard cheeses, which contain low levels of lactose. You should aways consult a doctor before changing a child's diet.

SEE ALSO

Allergies and hay fever	**78–79**
Abdominal pain	**92–93**
Vomiting, diarrhoea and constipation	**96–97**

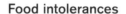

Common food allergens
Cow's milk, strawberries, peanuts, prawns and eggs are among the most common foods to trigger an allergy.

Your child's skin

The largest organ in the body is the skin. Sometimes the way the skin functions can go wrong, and this can create problems – especially in babies and young children whose skin is more sensitive than that of an adult.

Skin has a complex structure and performs several vital functions that are essential to survival and wellbeing. It forms a barrier that protects the internal organs from external elements such as bacteria and other infections, and has several components that help to regulate body temperature. Skin varies in thickness, depending on the area of the body it covers – for example, it is thinner on the eyelids than it is on the soles of the feet.

There are two main layers of skin: the epidermis and the dermis. The epidermis is the thin surface cover that you can see and is subdivided into three layers of cells. The innermost layer – the basal cell layer – contains living cells that constantly divide to produce new cells to replace ones worn away at the skin surface. This layer also contains the melanocyte cells, which produce the pigment melanin. It is melanin that gives the skin its colour and helps protect against sunburn. Above the basal cell layer is the intermediate, or prickle, cell layer. These cells can grow abnormally to form warts. The outer layer is made up of flat, dead cells composed of

Layers of the skin

The innermost layer of skin is the dermis, where the nerves and capillaries are found. The outer layer is the epidermis, essentially a protective covering.

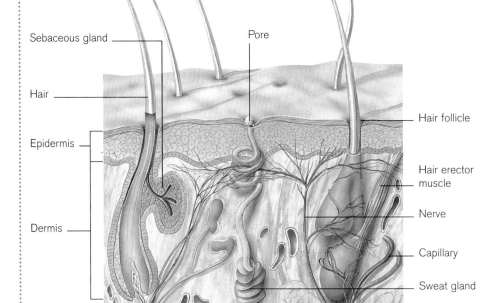

- Sebaceous gland
- Pore
- Hair
- Hair follicle
- Epidermis
- Hair erector muscle
- Nerve
- Dermis
- Capillary
- Sweat gland
- Subcutaneous tissue

keratin, a type of hard protein. They are constantly being shed and replaced by cells from the basal cell layer. The cells in the outer layer are cemented together by a fatty film, called the lipid layer, which forms a protective waterproof coating for the skin.

The dermis is the thick inner layer of the skin, which sits on top of fatty subcutaneous tissue. The dermis is made up of connective tissue that contains collagen (fibres of protein) and keeps the skin firm and supple. Many specialized structures, such as blood vessels, hair follicles, nerves, sweat glands and sebaceous glands, are contained within this layer.

The tiny blood vessels, or capillaries, assist the body's temperature regulation, as do the sweat glands, which produce perspiration. The sebaceous glands, which open into the hair follicles, make sebum, an oily sustance that lubricates the hair and forms a protective moisturizing film over the skin to help prevent it from drying out. The nerve endings and receptors in the dermis enable the skin to act as a receptor for certain sensations such as hot and cold, touch and pain.

A baby's skin

Although a baby's skin has many similarities to that of an adult, there are several important differences. At birth, a baby's skin is still developing and is five times thinner than that of an adult. It increases in thickness as the child grows, but the epidermis layer does not reach full maturity until puberty.

Because the sweat and sebaceous glands are immature and not fully functioning, the skin is a less effective barrier against infections, temperature and the environment. As a result, a baby's skin is more prone to dryness, irritation, spots and rashes. Production of the pigment melanin is slower, so the baby is more sensitive to the harmful effects of the sun's ultraviolet rays (see p.112).

Hair

Like the fingernails and toenails, hair is largely made up of dead cells containing keratin. The shaft of a hair rises above the surface of the skin, and its root is embedded in a hair follicle in the dermis.

There are three types of human hair. In the womb, lanugo is present on the foetus unitl about 36 weeks, when it is shed – but, sometimes, it is present on premature babies. After birth, vellus hair – a fine, short and colourless hair – covers most of the baby's body. Terminal hair is the long, pigmented hair that grows on the scalp, eyebrows and eyelashes. At puberty, vellus hair becomes terminal hair in the armpits and pubic area, as well as on the legs and, in boys, the arms and face.

The average daily hair loss is up to 100 hairs. More extensive loss of hair may be due to several causes, and it may be temporary or permanent.

SEE ALSO

Bathing your baby and helping him to sleep	**16–17**
Hair care	**42**
Infectious diseases	**60–61**

HOW SKIN PROTECTS

The skin protects against invasion of bacteria and other infections, physical injury, chemical pollutants, water loss and harmful ultraviolet rays. If the skin is damaged or broken, an infection may occur. If the fatty film (the lipid layer) is stripped away by an agent such as a harsh chemical or detergent, the skin will become dry and irritated.

The skin also protects by regulating body temperature, keeping the body warm in winter and cool in summer. If the body becomes too hot, the capillaries expand, causing more blood to flow to the skin surface and turning it red. The sweat glands then produce more sweat, which is mainly composed of water, salt and waste products. The evaporation of sweat on the skin has a cooling effect.

As the skin cools, or if the body gets cold, the capillaries contract to prevent the flow of blood to the skin surface and reduce heat loss. The skin then turns pale or looks white. Tiny hairs on the skin surface also help to maintain warmth by standing on end, with the help of hair erector muscles; the hairs trap air, which acts as insulation.

Eczema and dermatitis

The words "eczema" and "dermatitis" are often used interchangeably. However, eczema usually refers to a chronic dry skin condition, and dermatitis is used when the skin comes into contact with an irritating substance.

There are different types of eczema, but the most common one is atopic eczema, which affects up to 15 percent of children, regardless of their skin colour, and starts before the age of two. Patches of dry skin, which may crack or scale, appear on the face, behind the ears and knees, and in the folds of the neck and elbows. Eczema is not contagious, but an infection may result if the skin is damaged from scratching. The skin may become inflamed with pimples or blisters that erupt and weep – this is wet eczema.

Atopic eczema
The typical symptoms of atopic eczema are seen on this child's elbow – patches of dry, irritable, itchy skin.

The cause of eczema is unknown, but up to 70 percent of people with atopic eczema have a family history of eczema, asthma or allergic rhinitis. Other factors that have been implicated include chemical sprays, the droppings of house dust mites, pets, pollen, heavily perfumed products, soaps and biological washing powders. Hard water has been found to be one contributing factor in primary school children.

In some cases, certain foods may make the condition worse, but foods such as dairy products or wheat should not be eliminated from your child's diet without advice from your doctor or a dietitian (see pp.98–99).

Treating eczema

Currently, there is no cure for eczema, but 50 percent of children tend to be clear of the condition by the age of 2 and 90 percent by the age of 15.

Treatment should aim at keeping the eczema under control and minimizing any discomfort or itching. To keep your child's skin soft and moist, apply emollients or moisturizing creams several times a day. Avoid soap, bath preparations and irritants when bathing him. You can add emollients to the water for bathing; for some children, a tepid bath prepared with a capful of a children's nonperfumed bath oil brings relief. You should keep your child's nails trimmed (see p.43) to reduce the effects of his scratching.

Sometimes steroid creams are necessary for short periods to help the healing of badly damaged skin. Antihistamines may also be prescribed. In severe cases, wet wraps, in which moisturizers are applied to the child's skin before he is wrapped in layers of moist bandages, may be needed – a health care worker will teach parents how to apply the wraps.

Because the droppings of the house dust mite may be a trigger for eczema, keep furnishings to a minimum, and try to damp dust and vacuum when your child is out of the room. A wooden floor, ceramic tiles and vinyl or linoleum flooring are better than carpet. Limit the number of fluffy toys your child has in the cot or bedroom, and wash them once a week, along with the bedclothes, at 60°C (140°F) to kill any mites. Anti-allergy bedding may also help.

You should keep your child cool by making sure he wears cotton clothing and sleeps with cotton bedding. He should avoid excessive heating, an overly dry atmosphere and irritants such as perfumed washing products, chemical sprays and cigarette smoke – all of which can make eczema worse.

Contact dermatitis

Sometimes a rash appears when the skin comes into contact with an irritating substance. One form, allergic contact dermatitis, occurs when the body's immune system reacts against a substance such as the nickel in jewellery. Irritant contact dermatitis is another form, which occurs when the skin comes into contact with an irritating substance such as a harsh chemical or detergent. Your child should avoid coming into contact with the offending substance. If your child does touch it and gets a rash, calamine lotion or a paste made of bicarbonate of soda may help to soothe it.

Seborrhoeic eczema

Also known as seborrhoeic dermatitis, seborrhoeic eczema usually starts at about two months of age and appears on the scalp or as a rash in the nappy area. It can be confused with atopic eczema. The cause is unknown, but is thought to be due to a yeast infection. The condition usually looks far worse than it is and tends to trouble parents more than the child.

The scales may be similar to cradle cap (see box, below) or there may be a red, scaly rash, which can spread to the forehead, the eyebrows, behind the ears, the neck and the armpits. In the nappy area, the skin is red and flaky, with small white skin scales, and the rash may spread up the trunk.

In mild cases, treat the scalp in the same way as for cradle cap, but also bath your child daily with a nonsoap substitute and add oil to the water to loosen the scales and moisturize the skin. Pat the skin dry and apply a moisturizing cream several times a day. If the condition is severe or infected, a mild hydrocortisone cream, or a combination cream of hydrocortisone and an antifungal agent, may be prescribed by your doctor.

SEE ALSO

Asthma	**76–77**
Allergies and hay fever	**78–79**
Your child's skin	**100–101**
Noninfectious rashes	**110–111**

CRADLE CAP

If a baby has cradle cap, his scalp will be coated with white or greasy brownish yellow scales. It can occur soon after birth and is not usually seen after the first year. Cradle cap is harmless and is probably caused by overactive sebaceous glands. It looks unsightly, and it may spread to other areas of the body – where it is called seborrhoeic eczema or seborrhoeic dermatitis – but it will eventually clear of its own accord.

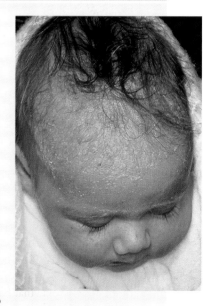

Until cradle cap clears, it can usually be removed by frequent gentle washing, using a mild baby shampoo or wetting the head and applying aqueous cream or emulsifying cream as a soap. To loosen the scales, aqueous cream or warmed oil can be massaged into the skin and left on for an hour or so, or overnight, before being washed off. In severe cases or if frequent shampooing does not work, a mild hydrocortisone cream may be prescribed by your doctor.

Birthmarks

About 1 in every 100 babies has some type of birthmark, either in the form of a skin discoloration or swelling. It may be present at birth or appear a few weeks later, and it may be permanent or temporary.

Also known as a naevus, a birthmark develops when there is an incorrect mixture of the pigment cells in the epidermis, the outer layer of skin, or there is an abnormality of the capillaries in the dermis, the inner layer of the skin.

The most common type of birthmark is the salmon patch, which is also known as a stork mark or stork bite. It is a flat, pink or red patch that is usually situated on the forehead, upper eyelid, bridge of the nose or the back of the neck. A stork mark is harmless and does not need treatment. Those on the face normally fade, but a mark on the neck may remain for life.

A proliferation of tiny, immature blood vessels can cause a haemangioma. The most common type is the strawberry mark, in which there are one or more raised red areas resembling a strawberry. It occurs in 1 in 20 babies, but is more common in girls and in premature babies. If the size or position causes problems, cryosurgery (in which tissues are destroyed by freezing) or other treatment may be needed.

A port wine stain is a flat, irregular area of the skin, usually on the face, neck or head, that is stained red or purple. It is caused by a malformation of capillaries in the skin. It is present at birth, grows with the child and does not fade. Rarely, port wine stains may be associated with Sturge-Weber syndrome, a congenital condition that can cause problems such as epilepsy. Pulsed dye laser treatment is a safe and effective treatment that benefits 80 percent of children with port wine stains.

A Mongolian blue spot is a bluish black area of skin that is seen on the lower back and buttocks of black and Asian babies, but it can occur in Caucasians. The spot, caused by a concentration of melanin cells deep in the skin, is present at birth. It will fade gradually, but may be mistaken for a bruise.

Strawberry mark

This type of birthmark develops during the first weeks of life, increases in size, then starts to shrink. Most disappear by the time the child is seven years of age.

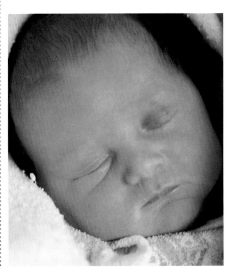

ERYTHEMA

The term erythema simply means redness of the skin, but it may be used as part of a description for other skin problems. A widespread erythema with malaise and fever is usually due to a viral infection or reaction to a drug.

Erythema toxicum is a common, harmless rash that affects half of all full-term babies in the early days of life. The rash consists of tiny bumps, surrounded by a ring of redness. Erythema multiforme is a rash with round, raised skin lesions, which can occur as a result of a viral or bacterial infection, especially herpes simplex (cold sore).

Bruises, blisters and boils

Although the skin is designed to protect the internal organs, it is not indestructible – it can be damaged, for example, by an accident or by an infection.

A bruise appears as a discoloured area of the skin and is caused by blood leaking from capillaries when the tissues under the skin are damaged. Children will get bruises in the course of everyday play and by accidental injury. Nonaccidental injury should be suspected if the bruising is severe, unexplained or in an unusual site. Bruising may also be caused by a bleeding disorder such as haemophilia.

To reduce the pain and swelling from bruises, you can hold a cold compress or ice pack on the area. You can also apply witch hazel or an arnica ointment.

Blisters

As a protective measure, fluid called serum collects between the dermis and epidermis of the skin, forming a blister. The most common cause of blisters is friction, such as when a shoe rubs against the heel. Blisters also occur from sunburn (see p.112), scalding or allergies. Rarely, blisters are the result of a skin disease caused by an immunological disorder.

You should never burst a blister, but you can cover it, if necessary, with a plaster or clean dressing. Small blisters are usually reabsorbed into the skin. Seek medical help for large or multiple blisters.

Boils

When an infection, most commonly due to the staphylococcus bacteria, starts in a hair follicle in the skin, a boil forms. It begins as a warm, tender, red lump that may throb. For several days it swells with pus and becomes more painful. As the boil gets bigger it forms a yellowish head, or centre, which eventually bursts through the skin. Once the pus escapes, the pain is relieved.

Do not squeeze the boil. Apply a hot compress, using cotton wool or a clean cloth soaked in hot water, several times a day to relieve the pain and hasten the bursting of the boil. If your child has repeated boils or a large boil, he should see a doctor. If the boil is ready to burst, the doctor may make a small cut in the centre to help the pus to drain. The doctor may also prescribe antibiotics to kill the bacteria. Recurrent boils can be a symptom of a disease such as diabetes (see pp.137–139) or anaemia (see p.116).

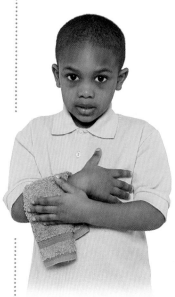

Treating a bruise
A flannel soaked in cold water makes an ideal compress for a bruise.

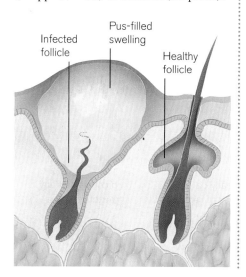

Infected follicle

Pus-filled swelling

Healthy follicle

How a boil develops
Bacteria enters a hair follicle and pus forms, blocking the hair. It is first recognized as a red, painful lump and soon forms a domed shape with a yellowish tip.

Acne

Acne is a skin disease characterized by spots. Its onset is usually at or just after puberty, but it may occasionally start at eight years of age. It can sometimes affect infants, in which case it is known as infantile acne.

In some cases, acne can persist into adulthood. Many teenagers suffer from acne, but there are several treatment options that can help minimize its effect.

Acne, which tends to run in families, is a disease of the sebaceous, or oil-producing, glands. It is a myth that acne is caused by foods such as chocolate or by poor hygiene. The oil, called sebum, is produced by the glands that normally

Severe acne

The red lesions on this child's back can be one sign – although not a welcome one – of a child entering puberty.

keep the hair and skin lubricated. The glands are controlled by the sex hormones called androgens. Increased production of sebum, which usually occurs around puberty, can cause blockage of the ducts through which the sebum normally passes. As a result, bacteria and dead skin cells build up, causing spots. The face is most commonly affected, but acne can also occur on the neck, back and chest.

Acne consists of several types of lesions, which may be inflamed or noninflamed, and they may be mild, moderate or severe, depending on the number and type of lesions present. Blackheads and whiteheads are noninflamed lesions. Blackheads, or open comedones, consist of a tiny plug of sebum and the skin pigment melanin – the black colouring is melanin, not dirt. Whiteheads, or closed comedones, are skin coloured. Inflamed lesions, which contain pus, are red spots (papules), yellow spots (pustules), nodules (large, deep, inflamed spots) and cysts (swellings filled with fluid).

A few comedones and spots, but little inflammation, is considered mild acne. More inflamed papules and pustules are moderate acne. Severe acne is when there are numerous pustules, nodules and cysts, which may leave scarring.

Treatment

A topical anti-inflammatory or antibacterial preparation, such as washes or gels containing benzoyl peroxide or retinoids (vitamin A derivatives), may be sufficient for mild acne. If these fail, topical antibiotics may be prescribed. Systemic antibiotics may be prescribed if topical antibiotics fail for moderate acne. A dermatologist may prescribe an anti-androgen and contraceptive preparation for females with severe acne. Oral isotretinoin, a powerful anti-acne drug, may be prescribed in severe cases, but it can have side effects.

Your child may need treatment for three months before there is any improvement. With severe acne, up to 12 months of treatment may be necessary.

Warts

Tiny lumps on the skin caused by one of the human papilloma viruses (HPV) can form into warts. They are common in children and are passed from person to person by close physical contact.

SEE ALSO

Feet and foot care	40–41
Infectious diseases	60–61
Your child's skin	100–101
Bruises, blisters and boils	105

The virus can enter the skin – and, in some cases, the mucous membranes – through cuts, scratches or cracks and incubate there for many months. It affects only the top layer of skin, the epidermis, causing a harmless, but rapid growth of skin. Warts do not have roots, but sometimes there may be one or more black dots in the wart, caused by capillaries that have become clotted because of the rapid skin growth.

There are several types of wart (see chart, right). Although they can affect any part of the body, they are most commonly found on the hands and feet. Warts are normally painless, except for plantar warts.

Treatment

Almost half of all warts will disappear without any treatment, however, they may take from a month to three years to do so. With the exception of plantar warts, there is no specific antiwart treatment. Topical applications, such as those containing salicylic acid, lactic acid or glutaraldehyde, are available from pharmacies and can be tried at home.

If the over-the-counter treatments fail, your doctor may freeze the wart with liquid nitrogen or other chemicals, a process known as cryotherapy; burn it off with electricity, which is referred to as cauterization; numb the skin and scrape it off, a process called curettage; or remove it using laser surgery.

Plantar warts (verrucas)

Children may pick up this type of wart by walking barefoot near swimming pools and in changing rooms. Pain may be caused when walking due to pressure, overlying hard skin, infection or inflammation of the wart.

Treatment includes applying a topical salicylic acid or lactic acid solution or gel, or a salicylic acid plaster, but the wart may take a few weeks to disappear. To help prevent spreading the virus, cover the wart with a verruca sock or waterproof plaster when your child goes swimming.

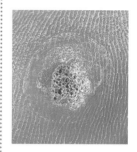

Plantar wart
This painful type of wart typically forms on the sole of the foot.

TYPES OF WART	
Name	**Description**
Plane warts	Small, flesh-, pink- or brown-coloured warts with flat tops. They usually occur in children on the face and back of hands. There may be multiple warts that grow in a line.
Common warts	Skin-coloured warts with a rough consistency; they are most common on the face and hands and several of them may join together.
Filiform warts	Long threadlike warts or skin tags; they may be seen on the face and neck.
Genital warts	This type of wart is transmitted by contact with another person carrying the virus. In children, it may be a sign of sexual abuse – you should seek advice from your doctor.
Plantar warts	Also called verrucas, plantar warts occur on the sole of the foot, usually on the weight-bearing area of the forefoot and heel.

Infectious rashes

Athlete's foot, herpes, impetigo, ringworm and scabies are all contagious infections that cause rashes. They may be caused by a virus, fungus or bacteria, but they are usually easily treated.

Athlete's foot is a common fungal infection that occurs among school-age children, as well as adults. It is particularly prevalent among older children, because they use communal changing rooms in gyms and swimming pools, and most movement and drama sessions within schools take place with the children barefoot.

If your child contracts athelete's foot, you should treat it as quickly as possible. Not only can it be extremely irritating and unpleasant for the sufferer, but it is also contagious and easy to spread to others – both to family members at home and to others in communal areas.

Herpes simplex is the virus that is responsible for neonatal herpes, genital herpes (usually in adults) and cold sores. It should not be confused with herpes zoster – the virus that is responsible for chickenpox (see p.63) and shingles. Cold sores from the herpes simplex virus are common in children and easily passed on through kissing and close contact.

Impetigo is a contagious bacterial infection that enters skin through a break, such as a cut or scratch, especially in

INFECTIOUS RASHES

Condition	Symptoms	Treatment/Prevention
Athlete's foot	The first indication of athlete's foot will probably be your child's complaints of itchy or sore feet – usually between the fourth and fifth toes. The skin will appear cracked and scaly and, if the condition has gone unnoticed for some time, it may be red and raw underneath.	Applying an antifungal powder will provide immediate relief and help the condition to clear up quickly, but you should also ensure that the rest of the family does not share the towel your child uses after bathing and that she only stands on her own bath mat while she dries herself. Excessive sweating aggravates this condition and trainers provide the ideal medium for the fungus to flourish. Buy socks with as high a cotton content as possible, and dust the inside your child's socks and shoes with the antifungal powder before she puts them on each day. Ensure that she baths regularly and dries between her toes carefully.

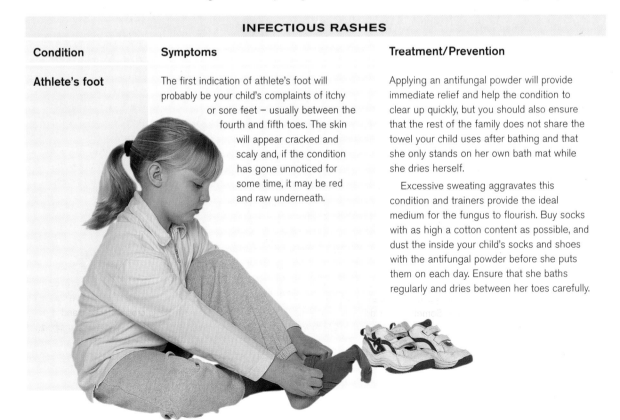

warm weather. If the child has existing skin problems, such as eczema, cold sores or urticaria, it can aggravate them.

Ringworm is a fungal infection that is no longer common, although it is infectious. Your child could contract it directly from an infected person, dog or cat, or from infected flakes of skin or hair if she comes into contact with them. Scabies, an irritating rash, is caused by the burrowing of minute mites, which are passed on from people and pets.

SEE ALSO

Feet and foot care	**40–41**
Infectious diseases	**60–61**
Your child's skin	**100–101**
Noninfectious rashes	**110–111**

INFECTIOUS RASHES

Condition	Symptoms	Treatment/Prevention
Impetigo 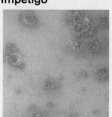	Impetigo is not difficult to spot because it has a very particular appearance. Small, red pimples appear first, usually around the mouth and nose, and they break down and weep to form yellow, brownish crusts. As the area heals, there will be reddened rings of skin around the outside of each crust.	The condition is easily and quickly cured by antibiotic ointment. If the outbreak is severe, the doctor may prescribe an oral medication as well. It is important to remember to wash your hands thoroughly after applying your child's ointment and to discourage her from touching the infection because it can be easily transferred to another area.
Herpes simplex (cold sores)	The first signs are small blisters in the mouth and on the lips, which sometimes turn to little ulcers. There may also be inflamed gums, a high temperature, swollen glands, a coated tongue and bad breath. None of these symptoms are serious unless they appear on a newborn baby or a baby already suffering from eczema.	Treat a cold sore as soon as it appears. It will feel itchy and irritating, and if your child scratches the sore, it could become infected and she could infect her eyes (see p.153). You can place an ice cube on the lips at the first sign of a sore, but creams, lotions and sticks that are formulated to reduce the risk of infection as well as ease the discomfort are available from a pharmacy. Cold sores can be recurrent; your child will be more prone to an attack if she has a cold, is run-down or is exposed to extremes of cold or heat.
Ringworm 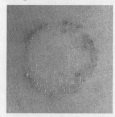	Ringworm is most common in the groin area, where it appears as circular, flaky patches, but it can also appear on the face or arms, or cause bald patches on the scalp. If the nails are infected, they become thick, distorted and discoloured.	This condition can be cured over time with an antifungal ointment and, if necessary, a course of antibiotics. It is vital to keep the bedlinen and towels your child uses separate from the rest of the family and to sterilize or throw away hairbrushes and combs that were used while she was infected.
Scabies	Scabies is easily detected – your child will feel very itchy and you may notice fine zigzag lines and blisters between her fingers and on her palms, wrists, elbows, armpits and trunk. Sometimes children suffer allergic reactions or develop a bacterial infection because of scabies.	Your child should see a doctor as soon as possible, who will prescribe a solution that should be applied everywhere except around the eye area. The whole family will have to be treated to avoid cross-infection, and if you have a pet, you should have it examined by a vet. After treatment, wash any bedding and clothing to ensure that you eradicate this nuisance quickly.

Noninfectious rashes

Skin rashes are not always from an infectious source. Sometimes they occur when the skin comes into contact with a particular substance such as soap. In some children, they may appear as a reaction to an allergen.

Nappy rash is a common problem for babies, especially when they are between the ages of 4 and 18 months. The rash is actually a form of contact dermatitis, and it is sometimes known as nappy dermatitis.

The main cause of the problem is a chemical reaction of the baby's skin to prolonged contact with urine and faeces, which can occur with both cloth nappies and disposable ones. Ammonia from the urine or bacteria from the faeces can burn or irritate the skin, which may then break open. The skin can be further irritated by friction from the nappy, which is created as the baby moves about.

Other possible irritants include chemical agents in the products that are often used to clean a baby's skin, such as strong soap, alcoholic wipes or bubble bath. Other chemical agents to avoid are biological washing powder or detergent used to wash the baby's nappies or clothes. If a baby is allergic to certain foods, a nappy rash may occur when he starts weaning (see p.35). Another type of dermatitis, seborrhoeic dermatitis, can also cause a nappy rash.

An allergic reaction

Urticaria is a common skin reaction, resulting in raised itchy red weals. There are other causes, but the main reason that this rash develops is usually a reaction to an allergen. As a result of the allergic trigger, the immune system makes IgE antibodies, which release histamine into the lower layers of the skin. Histamine dilates the tiny blood capillaries under the skin, which, in turn, leak fluid into the surrounding tissue, causing the rash.

Although there are many causes of urticaria, in 50 percent of cases the cause cannot be identified. However, people with asthma, hay fever or eczema are more susceptible to urticaria because they have an atopic disposition – they and other members of their family have a tendency to have allergic-based disorders.

Almost any medication – whether applied to the skin or taken by mouth – can cause an allergic reaction, although the most common drugs to do so are penicillin and aspirin. Iodine, which may be used to clean a wound or in certain medical tests, can also trigger an allergic reaction. Children who have had an allergic reaction to shellfish should avoid any medication or tests that use iodine.

Urticaria rash

The red weals typical of this rash are harmless but often cause irritating itching. Encourage your child to avoid scratching them, which can make the condition worse.

Sometimes an urticaria rash occurs when the skin comes into contact with an irritating substance, for example stinging nettles and other plants. This is more commonly referred to as nettle rash or hives.

Other common causes of urticaria include: foods such as strawberries, peanuts, milk, eggs and seafood; food additives such as tartrazine (E102); exposure to cold, sunlight, heat and pressure; and insect bites and stings.

SEE ALSO
Allergies and hay fever **78–79**
Eczema and dermatitis **102–103**
Food allergies and intolerances **98–99**

NONINFECTIOUS RASHES

Condition	Symptoms	Treatment/Prevention
Nappy rash	The rash can vary from a mild red patch on the bottom to angry looking, moist skin, with open spots, pimples or blisters all around the nappy area. The rash can become infected by the candida organism, or thrush, if the baby has a persistent nappy rash that does not clear up with ordinary nappy rash creams and the skin is bright red with white or red pimples in the folds. A thrush rash is more common in newborn babies and may occur if the mother has vaginal thrush. The baby may also have oral thrush (see pp.152–153).	Change a wet or soiled nappy as soon as you can, and clean the area with a mild soap or nonsoap substitute and water, oil or baby lotion. Do not use harsh baby wipes. Apply a nappy cream or calendula-based cream to protect and heal the skin. Avoid heavy barrier creams with disposable nappies; they clog the nappy and prevent the urine passing through. To help healing, leave the nappy off to expose your baby's skin to the air as often as you can. Use an antifungal cream for a candida rash. If you use cloth nappies, after sterilizing them, wash them in a nonbiological detergent and rinse well. Avoid using plastic pants – they prevent air from reaching the baby's skin.
Drug rash	The type of rash it causes and how long it lasts varies according to the medicine. For example, external contact with a drug such as an antibiotic cream or eye ointment may cause contact dermatitis (see p.103). Taking a drug by mouth or injection may cause itching or widespread urticaria (see below).	The rash will disappear once the drug is stopped. Calamine lotion or a paste made from bicarbonate of soda can help soothe it. Always inform a new doctor if you know that your child is allergic to certain drugs.
Urticaria	Individual red weals appear rapidly anywhere on the body and eventually become white or yellow with a red rim. The weals vary in size and number and are accompanied by severe itching, stinging or prickling. The rash may come and go over several hours, with new patches appearing as others disappear, but it usually disappears after 24 hours. In some cases, daily attacks can occur for months or years – this is known as chronic urticaria. Urticaria is usually a harmless but irritating condition for most people, but a few develop angio-oedema, in which there is swelling of parts of the body such as the face and eyelids. If the tongue or throat are affected, air may be prevented from reaching the lungs.	If there are symptoms of angio-oedema, seek medical help immediately. Otherwise, calamine lotion or a paste made from bicarbonate of soda can soothe the itch, and oral antihistamines can help shorten the length of attack. Prevention involves identifying and avoiding any factors known to trigger a reaction.

Sunburn

Children need a certain amount of sunshine – about 15 minutes a day – to help make vitamin D for strong bones, but overexposure can cause sunburn, which may increase the risk of skin cancer in later life.

A day outdoors

Keeping your baby covered up is the best preventative measure against sunburn. A parasol will also provide some protection.

A child is particularly vulnerable to sunburn because her skin is thinner than an adult's skin, and her body may not be able to produce enough of the tanning pigment melanin to protect her. Children with fair or red hair, blue eyes and freckles are more susceptible to sunburn than others.

In a case of mild sunburn, the skin will be red and sore. If there is severe sunburn, there can also be blisters and severe pain, and the child may develop sunstroke or heat stroke, which can be dangerous, even life-threatening.

Protection from the sun

Sunburn can occur even on a dull summer's day, whether your child is swimming or playing outside. Avoid exposing babies under the age of six months to direct sun and try to keep older children out of the sun between 11.00 am and 3.00 pm, when it is at its most dangerous. Don't let your child run about all day in a swimsuit or without any clothes on. In particular, protect her shoulders and the back of her neck; these are the most common areas for sunburn. Let her wear loose cotton clothes, such as an oversized T-shirt with sleeves, a floppy hat with a wide brim and sunglasses with an ultraviolet filter.

Apply sunscreen or sunblock often to any exposed parts of your child's skin. Use a preparation that has a minimum sun protection factor (SPF) of 15 and that protects against two types of ultraviolet radiation – UVA and UVB. If your child swims, use a waterproof sunblock.

If, in spite of all precautions, your child gets sunburnt, cool her with a tepid bath, shower or cold compresses, apply calamine lotion or aftersun cream, and give her cool drinks. If the sunburn is severe, or your child is feverish, vomiting or seems confused, consult your doctor.

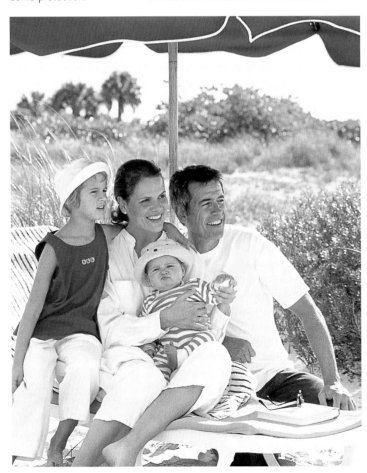

Hair problems

The most common hair problem that a child may have to contend with is head lice, which is no reflection on your standards of hygiene. Some children may experience hair loss, or alopecia, but this is usually not permanent.

SEE ALSO

Bathing your baby and helping him to sleep	**16–17**
Your child's skin	**100–101**
Infectious rashes	**108–109**

Children may suffer more than one attack of lice during childhood. Lice are insects that live on hair near the scalp and can be difficult to see. They are transmitted by close head to head contact and cannot jump or fly. They have usually been on the scalp for three or four months before the head itches. Nits are white, empty eggshells left after the lice have hatched. If you find lice on your child's head, the whole family and any close contacts should be treated, and you should inform her school.

Head lice treatment

Lice can be removed by wet combing or using insecticide lotions. Wet combing involves using a special comb to remove the lice. Comb over a sheet of white paper or when your child is in the bath so that the lice are more visible. Repeat the wet-combing routine every three to four days for two weeks so that any hatching lice can be removed before they lay new eggs.

Lotions containing insecticides, such as malathion, phenothrin, permethrin or carbaryl, can be used when lice are seen. Check with your doctor before using a lotion on a baby under six months old or if your child has asthma or eczema. Follow the instructions on the package carefully. If, after rinsing the product off, live lice are still on the head, or are seen a day or two after treatment, they may be resistant to the insecticide. Use the wet-combing method or switch to a product

with a different ingredient. (Products that contain phenothrin or permethrin belong to the same insecticide group.) Give a second application of the same treatment a week later. Do not use malathion- or carbaryl-based products more than once a week for three weeks at a time.

Concerns have been expressed about the toxicity of insecticides, and carbaryl is only available on prescription. Some parents use essential oils. If you use them, do so with caution – little research has been done on their toxicity. Use lotions or essential oils only when lice have been detected and never as a preventative measure.

Hair loss

A child may experience hair loss for several reasons. A baby may lose hair by rubbing her scalp against the mattress, as a type of headbanging, but she will usually grow out of this habit. It may also be caused by hair pulling, which may be done subconsciously and may be a sign of emotional distress. Patchy hair loss may be caused by hair styling such as ponytails and plaits.

Generalized hair loss may occur after exposure to drugs such as those used in chemotherapy, but the hair starts to grow back a few months after treatment ends. Alopecia areata, in which there·is patchy hair loss, may be associated with an autoimmune disease.

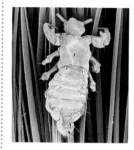

Head louse on hair
A louse, smaller than the head of a match, finds wet hair hard to cling to.

Wet-combing approach
After shampooing, leave a conditioner in. Use a normal comb, then comb through sections of the hair from the roots using a lice comb; wipe it clean between strokes.

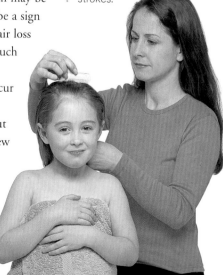

Heart, blood and circulation

The circulatory system carries red cells rich in oxygen, as well as white cells that help fight infection. It links to every cell in the body, exchanging nutrients for waste.

The circulatory system consists of a vast network of vessels with a pump – the heart – at its centre. The blood it pumps travels around the body in arteries with elastic yet muscular walls and is returned to the heart in less rigid veins.

Two arteries carry blood away from the heart: the aorta transports red, oxygen-rich blood and the pulmonary artery carries unoxygenated blood that has already travelled through the body to the lungs to be reoxygenated. Both arteries become smaller during their course and subdivide into arterioles and, finally, tiny capillaries. These form a fine mesh that permeates the tissues and provides access to every cell, allowing nutrients and waste products to be exchanged.

Arterial capillaries turn into venous capillaries within the mesh, and the blood within them then starts its journey back to the heart. It travels through ever-widening veins, which are consolidated into two main veins – the inferior and superior vena cava – which enter the heart.

Blood and its constituents

Blood has three main constituents: red cells, white cells and platelets. The carrier for all of them is plasma, a straw-coloured fluid that contains a variety of chemicals.

In an adult, there are about 5 litres (8¾ pints) of blood, containing 5 million red blood cells, or erythrocytes, in each cubic millimetre, which are replaced every 120 days. A one-year-old child has only 1 litre (1¾ pints) of blood. Erythrocytes are made in the bone marrow, and they contain the pigment haemoglobin, which combines with oxygen in the lungs to transport it around the body.

There are 4,000 to 10,000 white cells, or leucocytes, per cubic millimetre of blood. They perform a defensive function. The three main types are: lymphocytes, made in lymph tissue and bone marrow; granulocytes, formed in bone marrow; and monocytes, whose origin is unknown. Lymphocytes, monocytes and some granulocytes attack foreign bodies and make antibodies to combat them.

Platelets – of which there are 300,000 per cubic millimetre – make blood clot by

Bone marrow

Red blood cells are made in bone marrow. They start as stem cells, divide to form erythroblasts, then divide again to form red blood cells.

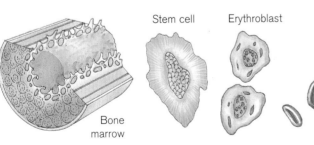

Bone marrow

Stem cell   Erythroblast

Healthy blood cell

THE LYMPHATIC SYSTEM

Another circulatory system found in the body transports excess tissue fluid – lymph. This fluid contains white blood cells and some chemicals that are also found in blood. Lymph helps fight infections and drains fluid from body tissues back into the bloodstream. The lymph permeates the body like blood does, but muscle movements, rather than a pump, make it circulate.

releasing chemicals that form a sticky mesh of protein, which attracts blood cells and then hardens.

The function of arteries and veins

A liquid similar to plasma, called tissue fluid, bathes each cell. In oxygenated blood, nutrients such as oxygen and glucose diffuse into the tissue fluid across the thin wall of the capillaries, and enter individual cells. At the same time, waste products from the cells' chemical activity, such as carbon dioxide, diffuse out of the cells and into the tissue fluid. From there, they enter the capillaries of the venous system to be returned to the heart.

The process is different in the blood carried in the pulmonary artery and its arterioles. This is deoxygenated blood, rich in carbon dioxide; it is pumped by the heart to the lungs. There, carbon dioxide is exchanged with oxygen before the blood is returned – reoxygenated – to the heart through the pulmonary veins, to be pumped through the aorta and around the body once again. It takes about 60 seconds for an erythrocyte to circumnavigate the body.

The circulatory mechanism

Blood is forced through the arteries by the pressure generated by the heartbeat – at 70 beats a minute in an older child – and the heart valves. The pumping phase, or systole, is created by the heart muscle contracting. The pressure should be at 90mm to 120mm of mercury (mm are units of measure based on early equipment that used mercury). When the heart fills with blood – diastole – the pressure is 60mm to 80mm. A typical reading would be given as 110/70. The pressure forces blood back to the heart through the veins, helped by the back pressure that draws blood into the heart's empty chambers.

The heart rate is higher and the blood pressure is lower in a younger child than it is in an older child.

Venous return is also assisted by muscles surrounding the veins, especially in the legs, which contract and squeeze the thin venous walls to force the blood upward. It cannot fall back because, unlike the arteries, the veins have one-way valves that prevent blood from returning.

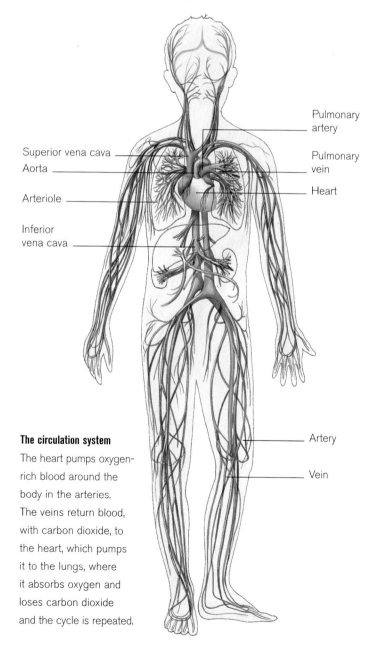

Superior vena cava
Aorta
Arteriole
Inferior vena cava

Pulmonary artery
Pulmonary vein
Heart
Artery
Vein

The circulation system

The heart pumps oxygen-rich blood around the body in the arteries. The veins return blood, with carbon dioxide, to the heart, which pumps it to the lungs, where it absorbs oxygen and loses carbon dioxide and the cycle is repeated.

Anaemia

A symptom, rather than a disease in itself, anaemia is the term used to describe a shortage or inadequacy of the red blood cells that carry oxygen around the body. It is the most common of all the blood disorders.

The deficiency of haemoglobin, which carries oxygen in the blood, is called anaemia. It has four main causes. The most common cause of anaemia, especially in childhood, is an insufficient amount of iron in the body to create adequate supplies of haemoglobin, which is made up of iron and protein. This is usually the result of an inadequate diet, a particular danger for vegetarian or vegan children and those who are fussy eaters. The problem does not usually occur until a child is at least 6 to 18 months old because babies are born with a supply of iron that lasts for the first six months of life.

Any infection can bring about mild anaemia because it reduces the efficiency with which the bone marrow produces red blood cells (see pp.114–115), as can, more seriously, any condition that affects the bone marrow directly. Leukaemia may affect red blood cell production (opposite). The production of red blood cells may also be affected by a lack of various chemicals that are vital to the process: vitamin B_{12}, because the body fails to absorb it; and folic acid and vitamin C due to an inadequate diet.

The loss of too much blood from the body, as a result of a serious wound, or from slow, regular bleeding, as in some disorders affecting the digestive tract, can also result in anaemia.

Haemolytic anaemia results from a condition in which red blood cells are destroyed such as in thalassaemia and sickle cell anaemia.

Recognizing the symptoms

The symptoms of anaemia include paleness, lethargy, headaches, dizziness, shortness of breath and general weakness. In addition, in the case of iron-deficiency anaemia, the tongue may be sore and the nails brittle. If untreated, the long-term effect may be impaired development of mental and physical functions.

Anaemia is primarily diagnosed by means of blood tests, and treatment is according to its cause. In the case of iron-deficiency anaemia, the doctor will recommend a diet with plenty of lean meat, liver, eggs and green vegetables, as well as an iron-rich milk formula and iron supplements.

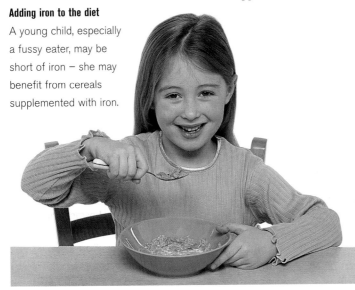

Adding iron to the diet
A young child, especially a fussy eater, may be short of iron – she may benefit from cereals supplemented with iron.

Leukaemia

A form of cancer, leukaemia occurs when too many white blood cells are made in the bone marrow and do not mature. Their sheer number impairs the production of healthy white blood cells, red blood cells and platelets.

SEE ALSO

Helping your child
in hospital   **56–57**

Heart, blood and
circulation   **114–115**

There are several forms of leukaemia, but the one that most often affects children is acute (that is, of sudden onset) lymphoblastic leukaemia; it accounts for 85 percent of cases. Other types that affect children are acute myeloid leukaemia and chronic myeloid leukaemia.

Leukaemia is the most common type of cancer to affect children. Its cause is not known, although exposure to radiation and viral infections are both suspected. The condition results in the huge number of immature, white blood cells leaving the body vulnerable to infection (see pp.60–61), especially to some potentially serious illnesses such as measles and chickenpox. The leukaemic cells also infiltrate organs such as the liver, spleen, lymph nodes and brain, which may affect their ability to function. Without medical treatment, leukaemia can be fatal within six months.

Symptoms

The symptoms of acute lymphoblastic leukaemia may include:
- Enlarged lymph glands, spleen and, sometimes, liver
- Anaemia
- Swollen joints
- Bruising, with pink or purple patches on the skin (petechia)
- A sudden high fever with a severe throat infection
- Nosebleeds
- Irritability.

Diagnosis and treatment

The diagnosis of leukaemia is made by blood tests and is confirmed by a biopsy of the bone marrow. Treatment is often in specialized centres and consists of chemotherapy for several weeks to destroy leukaemic cells. Blood transfusions may be necessary to combat anaemia and low platelet numbers.

In 90 percent of cases this treatment leads to a period of remission, when the symptoms of the disease disappear. Remission is confirmed by a biopsy of the bone marrow. Maintenance therapy with a number of drugs will continue for at least two more years after remission to prevent the condition from recurring. In at least 50 percent of cases, children are still in remission five years later.

A bone marrow transplant may be necessary in those cases that do not respond to treatment.

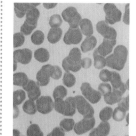

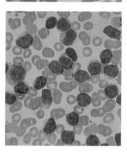

Blood cells

The top smear has a normal number of red blood cells; white cells predominate in the bottom smear.

HENOCH-SCHONLEIN PURPURA

Mainly affecting children between 5 and 11 years of age, Henoch-Schonlein purpura is an immune system disorder of unknown cause. It usually starts in the spring and is preceded by an upper respiratory tract infection. The first signs are a purple or pink rash, usually starting on the buttocks, which spreads. Arthritis then affects the joints, which swell, and there is abdominal pain with blood in the faeces and, sometimes, vomiting and diarrhoea. Eventually, the kidneys may be affected and there may be blood in the urine.

There is no specific treatment for the condition, but paracetamol may be given to relieve pain. However, in about 75 percent of cases, the symptoms clear up within a month or less. In some cases, there is a degree of damage to the kidneys.

Heart disorders

Congenital heart disorders – those that are present at birth – are not uncommon, and many clear up naturally over time without treatment. However, some can be life-threatening and require surgery to repair the heart.

Of every 1,000 babies born, between 6 and 8 of them will suffer from a heart defect, but the effects vary according to its seriousness. Many defects are minor and cause no problems; less serious defects can often be corrected by surgery. In extreme cases, congenital heart disorders can be fatal – they are responsible for the death of 10 percent of all babies who die during the first few weeks of life.

It is not fully understood why the heart develops incorrectly inside the womb. However, the risk of a heart disorder is increased if the baby has Down's syndrome or if the mother has untreated diabetes, if she contracts rubella (German measles) or takes certain drugs during the first three months of pregnancy (while her baby's heart is developing) or if she has had a previous baby with a heart disorder.

The heart normally has four chambers, two on each side of the septum. The upper chambers, the atria, fill with blood. Impulses from the heart's pacemaker trigger the muscles of the atrial walls to contract, forcing the blood through valves into the ventricle chambers. As the muscles relax, the valves return to their normal position, preventing any backflow of blood, and the ventricular muscles contract, forcing blood further through the system.

Types of heart defect

Broadly speaking, congenital heart disorders can be divided into two types: those in which, although there is an abnormality, the blood delivered to the body is fully oxygenated and those in which blood with reduced oxygen is directed to the body. Children in this latter category are often called blue babies because the lack of oxygen causes a bluish tinge to the skin (cyanosis).

Disorders in the first category include patent ductus arteriosus, in which the vessel that connects the pulmonary artery to the aorta in the foetus fails to close at birth; pulmonary stenosis, in which the

How the heart works

The right chambers of the heart pump deoxygenated blood to the lungs, while the left chambers pump oxygenated blood through the body.

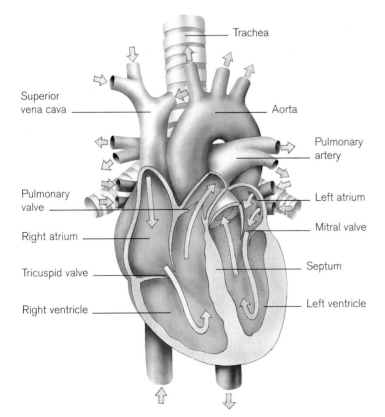

- Trachea
- Superior vena cava
- Aorta
- Pulmonary artery
- Pulmonary valve
- Left atrium
- Mitral valve
- Right atrium
- Tricuspid valve
- Septum
- Left ventricle
- Right ventricle

pulmonary valve is narrowed; aortic stenosis, a thickening of the wall of the aorta that impedes blood flow; ventricular septal and atrial septal defects (see box, below); and coarctation of the aorta, in which a portion of the aorta is narrowed, impeding blood flow. If these defects are severe, the child may need surgery.

Fallot's tetralogy is a combination of several heart defects. There is a ventricular septal defect (see box, below) and the aorta is displaced to the right. This is combined with a pulmonary stenosis, which results in the right ventricle becoming enlarged, or hypertrophied, in an attempt to compensate. A child with Fallot's tetralogy may develop cyanosis in the first year of life, depending on the severity of the condition; it is often apparent only as the child becomes more active and cannot cope with increasing physical demands. Surgery, in one or two stages, may take place when the child is between two and four years old.

Telltale signs

The symptoms of congenital heart disorders vary according to the severity of the disorder. In many cases, there may be few or no symptoms unless there has been physical exertion. Symptoms may include:
● A heart murmur – a swooshing sound that can be heard when a doctor listens to your child's chest. Murmurs frequently do not indicate a heart defect and can be heard in many children with normal hearts. In some cases, your doctor may decide that it is necessary to arrange for tests to exclude an abnormality.
● Difficulty experienced in sucking, breathing and eating.
● Fatigue and slow weight gain.
● Frequent respiratory infections.
● A bluish tinge to the lips and skin (the typical appearance of a blue baby).

Symptoms in an undiagnosed, older child include clubbing of the toes and fingers. He will often be breathless after exertion, so he may adopt a squatting position, with his knees drawn up to his chest to help regain his breath.

Seeking medical help

Heart defects are diagnosed by using X-rays, electrocardiograms (ECGs) and ultrasound heart scans. Many septal defects clear up of their own accord before the child reaches the age of five, but if they do not, or in more serious cases, the defect will be repaired surgically. Such operations have a high rate of success. The best time for surgery is before the child reaches school age. The child may have to undergo a temporary procedure before having open heart surgery.

Children with some forms of heart defect have an increased risk of contracting bacterial endocarditis – an infection that may seriously damage the heart valves – if bacteria enter the bloodstream. This may occur during surgery or dental treatment, and in these instances antibiotics are normally given beforehand as a precaution.

SEE ALSO

Helping your child
in hospital   56–57
Heart, blood and
circulation   114–115

VENTRICULAR SEPTAL DEFECT

The most common type of congenital heart disease, which accounts for about 25 percent of all cases, is an isolated ventricular septal defect (VSD). In another 10 percent of cases, ventricular septal defect is associated with other abnormalities of the heart. The two parts of the septum dividing the ventricles normally fuse before birth, but in this condition it fails to happen, leaving a hole between the two ventricles. A similar condition occurs when there is a hole in the septum between the atrium chambers – this is known as an atrial septal defect.

In most children with ventricular septal defect, the diagnosis is made by chance when a heart murmur is noted. Most children have no symptoms and the hole closes of its own accord. Occasionally, surgery is necessary if the hole does not close. Antibiotics should be given if the child needs dental treatment or any form of surgery.

Bones, muscles and joints

The human body is supported by a framework of bones – the skeleton. Movement is produced by muscles, which usually act on the bones that meet at joints.

At birth, the average number of bones in a baby's skeleton is 213; however, some of the bones fuse together and by adulthood the skeleton consists of an average of 206 bones. The skeleton protects the delicate internal organs and, surrounded and linked by muscle and connective tissue, provides the body's basic ability to move.

The skeleton starts to develop soon after conception as the foetus grows in the uterus. First, a fibrous mesh of proteins binds together to create a gel of water and chemicals. This is cartilage, a hard, yet pliant, substance that forms the gristle in meat. Columns of cartilage build up, growing at both ends and thickening as new sheets are laid down.

After seven weeks a process known as ossification starts. The cartilage in the centre of the columns degenerates, leaving holes behind that are filled with bone marrow, in which blood cells are made. Bone-producing cells then lay calcium down on the remaining cartilage, and a network of blood vessels spreads through it, supplying oxygen and nutrients. This central honeycombed area is known as spongy bone, and hard, or compact, bone is laid down outside it. The combination of the two prevents bone from weighing too much, but means that bones are more fragile and can break more readily.

By birth, only the ends of the bones – epiphyses – are still made of cartilage, and it is from them that future growth takes place. Growth continues until the end of adolescence, under the control of hormones, in a fairly precise way – an X-ray of an epiphysis shows the age of the bone. However, not all cartilage turns into bone. It persists inside joints and in the ears, nose and throat.

Joints

It is the joints, the junctions between bones, that make movement possible – without them, the body would be rigid and static. There are three types of joint: fibrous, cartilaginous and synovial. Fibrous joints, which knit the bones of the skull together, have fibrous tissue between the bones that does not allow movement. Cartilaginous joints, in which the bones are connected by a disc of fibrous cartilage, are found between the vertebrae of the spine and each allows a small range of movement.

Most joints in the body are the synovial type. The surfaces where two bones meet are lined with friction-reducing cartilage and the area is contained within a fibrous joint capsule. This is filled with synovial fluid, a lubricating, shock-absorbing liquid, and is strengthened by ligaments that run between the bones and around the joint. Bursae, hollow areas in and around the joint capsule, also contain synovial fluid and reduce friction between tendons and bones.

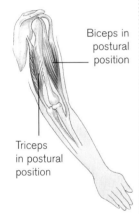

Biceps in postural position

Triceps in postural position

Contracted biceps

Relaxed triceps

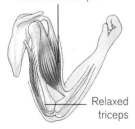

How muscles work
To raise the forearm, the biceps muscle in the upper arm contracts to move the forearm at the elbow joint. The triceps muscle in the lower part of the upper arm must relax and lengthen.

There are several types of synovial joint; each has a different range of movement. Hinge joints, for example, only allow movement in one plane, like the hinge of a door – the main ones are at the knee, ankle and elbow. Ball and socket joints at the shoulders and hips allow a wider range of movement because the ball-like head of one bone rotates in three dimensions within the socket of another bone.

Muscles

The muscles have two main functions: they maintain posture and contract and relax to move bones within joints. Babies are not born with enough control over their muscles to allow them to stand and move. They must learn control and coordination – this starts from the head with their neck muscles, and continues downward to their torso and legs.

The end of each muscle is anchored to bone by means of a tendon, a strong band of fibrous tissue. When a muscle contracts, the bone is moved in its joint by the tendon. However, another muscle, or group of muscles, must relax and lengthen. The contracting muscle is taking action – it is the agonist. The relaxing muscle is the antagonist. For every agonist there are one or more antagonists.

A muscle is not always taking direct action. For example, when the forearm is held out to the side, both the triceps and the biceps maintain a degree of tension to help hold the position. In this case they are acting as postural muscles, being neither agonists or antagonists.

Muscles are made up of bundles of fibres that are composed of smaller fibres, or filaments. Some of the filaments are thicker than others, and when a muscle contracts, the two sizes of fibre slide in on each other, shortening each cell and so shortening the muscle.

The types of fibre within a muscle depend on that muscle's function. Muscles whose main purpose is to maintain posture contain mostly slow-twitch fibres, which are red in colour and contract slowly and repeatedly over a long period. White, fast-twitch fibres contract quickly in short bursts and are found mostly in muscles used for quick, decisive action. The fibres in muscles can tear, but will usually heal.

SEE ALSO

Heart, blood and circulation	**114–115**
Muscular aches and pains	**122**
Sprains and strains	**123**

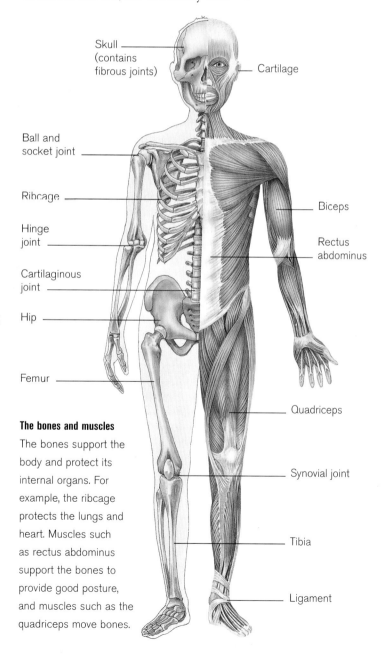

Skull (contains fibrous joints)

Cartilage

Ball and socket joint

Ribcage

Hinge joint

Cartilaginous joint

Hip

Femur

Biceps

Rectus abdominus

Quadriceps

Synovial joint

Tibia

Ligament

The bones and muscles
The bones support the body and protect its internal organs. For example, the ribcage protects the lungs and heart. Muscles such as rectus abdominus support the bones to provide good posture, and muscles such as the quadriceps move bones.

Muscular aches and pains

Children are not as susceptible to muscular aches and pains as most adults are, but some children can experience back pain and muscle cramps.

Cramps can be very painful, but they are not dangerous. They are caused by the sudden and involuntary contraction of a muscle or group of muscles that then fail to relax. Precisely why this happens is not known, but cramps often follow unaccustomed, strenuous or repetitive exercises, and they have been associated with a reduction in the levels of salts in the body as a result of excessive sweating or diarrhoea.

The best way to relieve a cramp is to stretch the affected muscle. In the calf, for example, have your child point his toes down as hard as possible and hold the position; then pull the toes up toward the kneecap and hold. He should repeat this until the cramp passes. Then apply heat with a hot water bottle wrapped in a towel or by giving him a hot bath or shower.

Preventive measures include:
- Making sure that your child performs a warm-up routine before taking exercise.
- Making sure that he takes plenty of fluid before, during and after exercise.
- Encouraging your child to take a hot bath after exercise to relax the muscles.

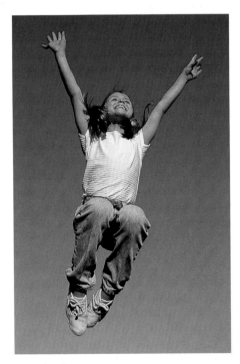

Natural exuberance

Many children are very active. To avoid painful cramps, make sure she drinks plenty of fluids when participating in a sport.

BACK PAIN

Two of the most common causes of back pain in adults are poor posture and osteoarthritis – the wear and tear that takes its toll on joints as a result of the ageing process. However, most children have naturally good posture and are too young to suffer from osteoarthritis, so back pain is rarely a problem for them – although it sometimes does occur.

Occasionally, back pain develops at the start of puberty. Sometimes this is because of a tendency for adolescents to adopt a slumped posture. Occasionally, the cause may be a condition known as Scheurmann's disease, in which the bone and cartilage in the spine become inflamed. The resulting pain typically lasts for between six months and three years and its severity varies considerably. The problem usually clears up when the child has finished growing.

If your child suffers from back pain frequently, you should consult your doctor so that any underlying disorder may be treated. Whatever its cause, back pain is treated by postural training, special exercises, rest and, in severe cases, physiotherapy.

Sprains and strains

A sprain affects a joint; it occurs when one or more of the ligaments that bind the joint together are overstretched or torn. A strain, or pulled muscle, occurs when some of the fibres in the muscle are overstretched or torn.

SEE ALSO
Bones, muscles
and joints   120–121
Muscular aches and pains   122
Broken bones   218–219

The direct cause of a strain or sprain is usually a fall, a sudden jolt, a sudden twist or a strenuous physical activity. Sprains and strains are rare in toddlers, whose joints and muscles are still extremely pliable. They are more of a risk when children start school and become increasingly active, and also in older children who are unfit and only take exercise irregularly. However, the majority of cases are mild and clear up naturally within a few days without any medical intervention being necessary.

Symptoms of both sprains and strains include local swelling, tenderness and pain on movement, a limp if the muscles or joints involved are in the leg and, if tissues have been torn, there may be bruising after a few days.

Treatment

The best treatment for strains and sprains is encapsulated in the acronym RICE:
- R is for rest. Avoid using the affected joint or muscle as much as possible.
- I is for ice. Cover the affected area with a cold compress such as crushed ice, a freezer pack or a bag of frozen peas wrapped in a tea towel to avoid an ice burn. Leave the compress in place for 5 minutes in the case of a toddler, for 15 minutes for an adolescent. Repeat two to three times a day for the first two days.
- C is for compression. Bandage a torn muscle or joint to give it support and prevent further swelling. Make sure that it is not too tight, otherwise you might restrict blood flow to the extremities.
- E is for elevation. Use a support to raise the affected area to help reduce swelling and aid the flow of fluids away from it. If the foot or knee is involved, for example, it should be raised above the level of the hips.

Frequent exercise, preceded by a warm-up routine and followed by cool-down exercises, is the best preventive measure.

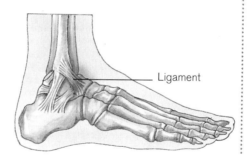

Ligament

Spraining the ankle

The ankle is a complex joint with a number of ligaments (for clarity, only a few are shown). It is one of the most common joints to be sprained.

OSGOOD-SCHLATTERS' DISEASE

The tendon attached to the thigh muscles joins the kneecap to form the patellar tendon. This tendon joins a bony protruberance – the tibial tubercle – which forms the growing point at the top of the shin bone. In Osgood-Schlatters' disease, both the patellar tendon and the tubercle become strained as a result of overuse of the thigh muscles during a time of growth. Adolescent boys are primarily affected, particularly those who are keen on sport.

The symptoms are pain, which increases with movement, localized swelling and sometimes a limp. Treatment consists of mild painkillers such as paracetamol or ibuprofen, ice packs and rest. Sport and exercise should be avoided when pain is present; in severe cases, immobilization may be necessary. The disorder usually cures itself with time, generally before adulthood.

Juvenile arthritis

Also known as Still's disease and juvenile rheumatoid arthritis, juvenile arthritis is a rare condition that affects about 1 child in every 6,500 each year. In 50 percent of cases, the problem resolves itself before adulthood.

The cause of juvenile arthritis is a malfunction of the immune system, which provides the body's defence against disease. Normally, this system attacks foreign matter that it perceives to be a threat, but when it malfunctions, some of the body's own cells are regarded as a threat and are attacked. It is not known why this happens. However, because juvenile arthritis tends to run in families, it is thought that there may be a genetic predisposition to it.

The result of the immune response is inflammation of the synovial lining of the joints and tendons, causing pain, stiffness and swelling and restricting mobility. The condition has acute and inactive phases, and it often dies out completely after being active for months or, sometimes, years. Depending on how long an acute phase lasts, there may be significant damage to the synovial linings, as well as to the underlying cartilage, bone and tendons. Any joint that has been damaged by juvenile arthritis is more susceptible to osteoarthritis in later life.

Types of juvenile arthritis

There are three types of juvenile arthritis, and they all have the same cause. Pauciarticular arthritis is the most common form, accounting for about half of all cases of juvenile arthritis. Girls under the age of eight are most susceptible. Generally, up to four large joints, such as the hips and knees, are affected, and some affected children have a special sero-positive antibody in their blood that is linked to an 80 percent increase in the risk that eye problems will also develop.

Polyarticular arthritis accounts for about 30 percent of cases. Five or more joints are affected – usually, although not exclusively, corresponding joints in both hands – for example, the same knuckles in the same fingers – or feet. This type of juvenile arthritis normally clears up spontaneously unless children – most likely girls – have the rheumatoid factor antibody in their blood. In such cases, the condition is similar to adult rheumatoid arthritis and is more severe.

Systemic arthritis, or Still's disease, the third type of juvenile arthritis, accounts for about 20 percent of cases. It normally develops in early childhood. Its onset is marked by a high temperature, enlarged lymph glands and spleen and a vague, transient pink rash that does not itch. The joints may either become swollen within days of the onset of this illness or after a few weeks.

Arthritic hands

Swollen finger joints are typical of polyarticular arthritis, in which the same joints are affected in both limbs.

SEE ALSO

Helping your child
in hospital   **56–67**

Bones, muscles
and joints   **120–121**

HOW YOU CAN HELP

It is vital that both family and friends help to make sure that a child with juvenile arthritis keeps as much independence and mobility as possible. Treat your child as normally as you can, avoid being overprotective and encourage social activities within her peer group.

During times of remission, encourage sport and physical activities – these are especially useful because they will help your child strengthen her muscles and maintain and improve the range of movement at joints.

Making a diagnosis

The diagnosis of juvenile arthritis and the identification of the type involved is made by the doctor after noting the signs and symptoms present in the child, checking for any family history of the disorder and testing the child's blood for the presence of autoantibodies and the rheumatoid factor. Other disorders that affect the joints such as an infection are ruled out.

Typical symptoms of the condition include swollen, red joints that are painful, especially after exercise and often when waking from sleep. The skin over the affected joints often feels warmer than usual.

Treating juvenile arthritis

There is no cure for juvenile arthritis, and treatment is aimed at reducing symptoms. Depending on their severity and duration, the following treatment may be advised:

● The child should rest, especially during an acute attack, with the inflamed joints supported by light splints. Physiotherapy may reduce stiffness and help mobility.

● Medication can be effective. Aspirin is not often prescribed for young children because of possible side effects (see p.63). Instead, nonsteroid anti-inflammatory drugs (NSAIDs), such as ibuprofen, may be used. Gold salts, penicillamine or methotrexate may be given as second-line drugs if NSAIDs are not effective, but it takes several weeks to see if they work. Steroids are avoided wherever possible because of their side effects, but they may be necessary in severe cases. Occasionally, local steroids such as hydrocortisone may be injected into a swollen joint to give temporary relief.

● Surgery to remove the thickened synovial sheath surrounding a joint or tendons may relieve pain and release trapped nerves. Ruptured tendons may also be repaired to maintain mobility and prevent deformities. In cases of severe disability, it may be necessary to replace a joint.

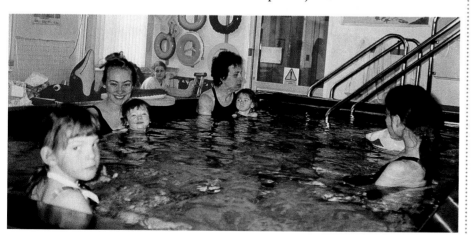

Hydrotherapy
Exercising in water can maintain muscle tone by taking the pressure off the joints, making them easier and less painful to move.

Muscular dystrophy

The term muscular dystrophy covers a number of different conditions in which the muscles waste away, and all of them are serious, inherited disorders. The most common form is Duchenne muscular dystrophy.

In Duchenne muscular dystrophy, a condition that principally affects boys, the gene responsible for the disorder is linked to the male X chromosome. It occurs in about 1 in every 3,000 baby boys and usually becomes apparent between the ages of three and six. The first signs are weakness in the pelvis and legs, which then spreads to the shoulders. One typical indication of Duchenne dystrophy is a child's habit of waddling – rather than walking – using his arms for leverage to help get up off the ground and having difficulty climbing stairs.

Keeping active
The goal in treating muscular dystrophy is to maintain the child's mobility and independence as much as possible.

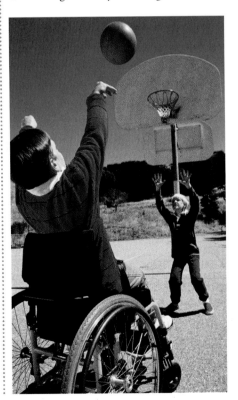

The level of disability increases as the muscles become weaker; most affected children have to use a wheelchair by the age of 10. The condition continues to deteriorate and it is unusual for someone with it to reach 30 years of age.

Other forms

The less common, and also less severe, forms of muscular dystrophy include:
● Becker dystrophy: occurs in 1 in every 60,000 births. It has the same, but less severe, symptoms as Duchenne dystrophy; those affected often live into middle age.
● Facio-scapulo-humeral dystrophy: attacks both girls and boys and can appear at any age, causing weakness in the face muscles, which spreads to the shoulders, then the pelvis. There are often periods of remission, so those affected have a much longer life expectancy than in other forms.
● Limb girdle dystrophy: appears from late childhood to early middle age and progresses slowly; it is eventually disabling.
● Emery-Dreifus dystrophy: appears in childhood to early adolescence; it slowly affects the shoulders, upper arms, shins and joints, and it may affect the heart.

Treatment

There is no treatment that stops the muscle wasting or cures it. Treatment consists of physiotherapy, hydrotherapy and the use of orthopaedic aids. Any deformity caused by the condition, such as scoliosis, may be corrected by surgery.

Scoliosis

The spine normally runs in a straight line up the back. However, sometimes it curves abnormally, either to one side or the other – although usually to the right. The curve is known as a scoliosis.

On rare occasions, the condition is present at birth, as a result of a deformity of the muscles or vertebrae. Occasionally, too, scoliosis is caused by another medical condition such as muscular dystrophy (opposite). It is not due to poor posture and the exact cause of the disorder is usually not known.

Scoliosis typically appears for the first time in an adolescent, usually a girl. Along with the curve in the spine, the child's shoulders may not be level and the chest may be more prominent on one side than on the other.

If you suspect your child has scoliosis, consult a doctor, who will monitor him by taking measurements to see if the condition is improving or deteriorating. A child with mild scoliosis may benefit from physiotherapy to help improve posture. If the scoliosis is progressive, treatment with a brace may stop the progression; however, in severe cases surgery may be necessary.

SEE ALSO

Helping your child
in hospital   **56–57**

Bones, muscles
and joints   **120–121**

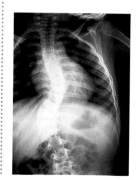

Spinal curvature

The curve in the spine of a young child with scoliosis is clearly visible in this X-ray.

Perthes' disease

The growth of bone depends on a good supply of blood to the epiphyses, or ends of the bones. In Perthes' disease, the blood supply to the head of the femur is inadequate; the reason is unknown. The area of bone breaks up, creating problems with movement and severe pain. If the condition is not treated, the femur may become permanently deformed.

Perthes' disease affects boys four times more often than girls. It usually appears between the ages of 2 and 10, with the incidence peaking between 4 and 6 years.

The symptoms of Perthes' disease include a stumbling, lurching gait with a limp and pain in the hip or knee. Consult your doctor immediately if your child shows these signs.

X-rays are used to make a diagnosis and monitor the condition. In mild cases, the pain may be relieved and the problem resolved by a few weeks' bed rest, although traction is sometimes necessary. In serious cases, a splint may be fitted, and in cases so severe that hip deformity is a risk, surgery may be needed to refix the head of the femur in its socket. The condition often clears up of its own accord within two years, but there is an increased risk of osteoarthritis later in life.

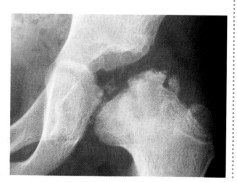

Deteriorated bone

The damage to the head of a femur in a six-year-old child with Perthes' disease can be seen in this X-ray.

Limping

Rather than a disorder in its own right, limping is a symptom of an underlying problem, and the cause is usually obvious – a blister, a splinter in the sole of the foot, ingrown or overlong toenails, badly fitting shoes or a strain or sprain in the foot.

If limping is persistent and has no obvious cause consult your doctor. Underlying problems that should be treated promptly include:
- A fractured bone or dislocated joint
- A slipped femoral epiphysis (the growing end of the thigh bone)
- Cerebral palsy (see p.169)
- A joint or bone problem, such

as juvenile rheumatoid arthritis (see pp.124–125) or a joint infection
- Perthes' disease (see p.127)
- Osgood-Schlatters' disease (see p.123)
- Congenital hip dislocation (opposite)
- Legs of unequal length.

If your child has a high temperature, a rash or a swollen joint, as well as a limp, consult your doctor straight away – there may be a bone or joint infection that requires immediate attention.

Most limps disappear when their cause has been treated, but a few, such as those caused by legs of unequal length, may require long-term treatment such as wearing specially adapted shoes.

Bow legs

An extremely common condition during a child's first two years of life is bow legs – in fact, bow legs are so common that they are not considered to be a disorder. In bow legs, also known as genu varum, the knees and lower legs are bowed outward.

The most common cause of legs forming into a bow is the position of the baby's legs as she grows in the womb. Generally, there is no underlying disease. However, there may be a different underlying cause in unilateral bow leg, in which only one leg is affected, and in severe or persistent cases of bilateral bow legs, where there is is a gap between the knees greater than 8 cm (3 in) when the ankles are placed together. Possible causes include:
- A previous fracture of the lower part of the femur (the thigh bone) or the

upper part of the tibia (the shin bone) that has not healed properly
- Juvenile arthritis (see pp.124–125)
- Rickets (a rare bone growth disorder caused by a vitamin D deficiency)
- Uneven growth at the epiphyses (see pp.120–121) caused by a previous fracture or injury or a bone infection.

Normally, the legs gradually straighten as the child develops and grows and begins to walk, so treatment is usually not necessary. However, you should consult a doctor if your child's legs do not straighten, if the condition becomes worse rather than better or if only one leg is bowed. In such cases investigation is by means of X-rays and blood tests and the underlying cause of the problem is treated. On rare occasions, the child may require surgery or have to wear braces to straighten the legs.

Baby legs

The outward curve of the lower legs is the obvious symptom of bow legs.

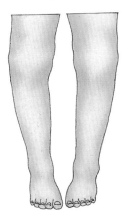

Knock knees

Like bow legs, knock knees – also known as genu valgum – are common in childhood. They occur when the knees are angled inward with the shin bones angled out. The cause of knock knees is not known, but it is common in children between the ages of three and four. The condition normally corrects itself by the time a child is 10 years old.

Treatment is necessary only if there is 8 cm (3 in) between the ankles when the knees are placed together and knock knees continue into adolescence. It takes two forms: either the growth of bone on the inner side of the epiphyses is slowed by stapling growth plates together or a small part of bone from the lower, inner side of the femur (the thigh bone) or the upper, inner side of the tibia (the shin bone) is removed.

Splayed legs

The classic sign of knock knees is feet that are splayed, even though the knees are touching each other.

SEE ALSO
Your newborn baby   **14–15**
Routine health contacts   **30–31**
Bones, muscles
and joints   **120–121**

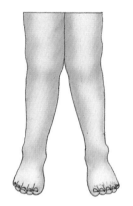

Congenital hip dislocation

In about 1 in 250 births, one or both hips dislocate – that is, the ball of the femur (the thigh bone) slips out of its socket in the pelvis – during birth or immediately after it. The cause may be a breech birth, an inherent weakness of the muscles at the hip, a shallow socket or looseness of the ligaments around the hip joint. The condition tends to run in families and affects more girls than boys.

Congenital hip dislocations are usually discovered during a routine health check immediately after birth or during the first year. The affected hip does not splay out freely when pushed, but gives a sudden jerk. With early detection, treatment is usually successful and the baby develops normally with no aftereffects. However, if the dislocation is not evident until the child tries to walk, treatment is more difficult and there is a risk that the child will have a permanent limp and be susceptible to osteoarthritis later in life. Symptoms in a toddler are limping, favouring the unaffected leg and extra skin folds on the buttock of the affected leg.

In a baby, a splint is applied for as long as necessary, which may be some months. In severe cases, traction may be required for a month before the splint is applied. In toddlers, traction is needed before a cast is applied. An operation may also be necessary to move the head of the femur into the correct position.

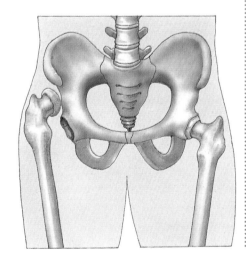

Dislocated hip

The ball of the femur in a normal joint (left) sits comfortably in the socket in the hip; in a dislocated hip (far left), the ball is separated from the socket.

Flat feet

In an adult's foot, the heel and the toes should touch the ground, but the area in between them should be raised off the ground, forming a flexible bridge that consists of three arches. If a person's arches fail to develop, or fall after they have developed, he is said to have flat feet, which are also known as fallen arches, or pes planus.

All babies have naturally flat feet because the arches do not fully develop until about the age of eight. The arches are also covered by an extra pad of fat. In some children – and the condition is common – the arches fail to develop; this may happen as a consequence of knock knees (see p.129) or be an inherited tendency. The first sign that parents notice is often an apparent weakness of the ankles, which seem to be turning in because of the way the feet are placed.

In most cases, flat feet do not cause any problems in childhood, even when the child is playing sport, and treatment is not necessary. However, in a small number of cases, the child will feel some pain and you should consult a doctor. Depending on the severity of the condition, he may recommend balancing exercises, physiotherapy and shoes with special pads that support the arches.

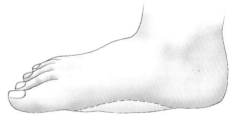

Flat feet
A baby's feet have extra fat, so they often appear flat. If you gently pull back the big toe, you will see a slight arch in his instep.

In-toeing

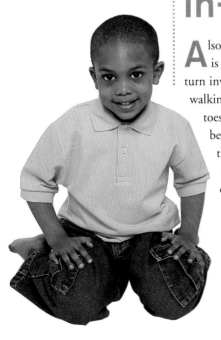

Also known as pigeon toes, in-toeing is a condition in which the toes turn inward when a child is standing and walking. Some babies start to turn their toes in when they begin standing between 8 and 15 months because their hips are curved inward and their legs are following the angle of the hip rotation. Another cause of in-toeing is the inward curving of the front part of the foot.

Generally, no treatment is necessary for in-toeing. If the cause is curved feet, they should correct themselves before the child is four years old. A hip rotation problem normally corrects itself by the time the child is eight years old.

However, in severe cases, in which the condition causes problems with balance, medical intervention may be required. Treatment may require the child to wear a splint at night, but doctors are often reluctant to advise such drastic measures. Instead, they may suggest physiotherapy and specially designed exercises.

Comfortable sitting
A child with in-toeing may be comfortable sitting in the W position, with his bottom resting on the ground between his legs.

Talipes

More commonly known as club foot, talipes is a congenital abnormality – that is, it is present at birth – and it occurs in 1 in every 1,000 babies. There are different types of club foot.

SEE ALSO

Helping your child
in hospital   **56–57**

Bones, muscles
and joints   **120–121**

One of the two most common types of club foot is talipes calcaneo-valgus. In this form of club foot, the heel rests on the ground, the toes turn up and the sole turns outward. Talipes calcaneo-valgus is generally caused by pressure placed on the baby's foot while it is in the womb, and usually only one foot is affected – this condition is known as a postural deformity.

Treatment for babies with talipes calcaneo-valgus starts immediately after birth and consists of a series of gentle stretching manipulations – in which the bones are manually repositioned – and exercises, and parents are taught to administer them to their child. These usually correct the problem, but in severe cases, it may be necessary for a surgeon to perform a manipulation at the age of one month and for the corrected foot to be kept in plaster for some weeks.

Talipes equino-varus

The most common type of club foot is talipes equino-varus. It occurs when the foot turns down and the sole is turned inward. It may run in families and is two to three times more common in boys than in girls. Both feet are involved in 50 percent of cases. In most instances, the cause is due to the way the baby was lying in the uterus before birth.

Talipes equino-varus usually resolves without treatment or physiotherapy. However, if the foot does not move to a normal position, the condition is more serious and active treatment will be necessary. The first step is a sequence of manipulations – sometimes one a week for five or six weeks – with the foot, or feet, being held in position between manipulations by splints, plaster of Paris or bandages. After three to four months, an operation may be needed to correct the abnormalities in the arrangement of bones, joints and muscles, and, again, the feet will be immobilized, this time for several months.

In severe cases, a series of operations may be necessary with the final one being delayed until after the child reaches the age of 12, when early growth of the foot has finished. In some extreme cases, it may be necessary for the bones of the foot to be broken and reset in a series of operations, between which the affected foot may be kept in position by means of adjustable metal cages.

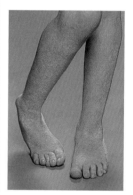

Club foot

Talipes equino-varus, in which the foot is turned down, can require years of treatment in a severe case, but the child will appreciate the results.

TOE-WALKING

Babies often walk on their toes when they learn to walk, but the habit is usually lost by the time they reach the age of two. Even at that age, occasional toe-walking is quite common. However, if a toddler toe-walks too much of the time, or only toe-walks, you should consult your doctor.

In some cases, the habit is associated with another condition such as cerebral palsy (see p.169) – albeit a mild form. Occasionally, medical treatment may be required. This normally involves confining the foot and ankle in a cast made of plaster of Paris for a month or so; it is usually successful.

The glands and hormones

Many of the body's functions are controlled by hormones, chemical messengers secreted by glands. These help regulate many processes in the body, including growth.

Throughout our lives hormones control a host of different processes. In childhood they are particularly important in helping the body grow and develop. Hormones also help maintain the chemical balance of the blood, help digest food, regulate the chemical activity of other cells (the metabolism), marshal the body's defences against stress and, in adulthood, enable us to reproduce. Both too much and too little secretion of hormones by the glands can lead to illness.

There are two main types of gland in the body: endocrine and exocrine. Endocrine glands, such as the thyroid, the adrenals and the gonads, are responsible for manufacturing and releasing most of the body's hormones, which travel around the body in the bloodstream. One key characteristic of hormones is that they are capable

The endocrine glands

The pituitary and other endocrine glands release hormones into the bloodstream, where they are transported to other organs and tissues.

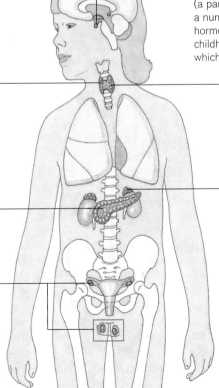

Thyroid gland: this gland produces hormones to control the heart and metabolic rate and, in children, to promote growth and development.

Pancreas: insulin is made in this gland, as well as the hormone glucagon, which stimulates the liver to produce glucose. Certain cells in the pancreas also secrete digestive hormones, or enzymes.

Gonads: starting at puberty, in girls the ovaries produce the hormones oestrogen and progesterone, which control the menstrual cycle and reproduction. In boys the testes produce the male sex hormone testosterone.

Pituitary gland: located below the hypothalamus (a part of the brain), this gland produces a number of hormones. These include a hormone that is involved in growth during childhood and ADH, antidiuretic hormone, which controls the amount of urine made.

Parathyroid glands: two pairs of tiny glands located behind the thyroid, they produce PTH, or parathyroid hormone, which regulates calcium in the bones. Calcium is important in children to ensure their bones grow.

Adrenal glands: found above the kidneys, these glands make adrenaline and noradrenaline, which regulate heart rate, blood pressure and the body's response to stress.

of affecting target cells that are some distance away from the gland that produces them.

Exocrine glands, such as the sweat glands and salivary glands, release their secretions directly into ducts or tubes, where they act locally on a nearby organ or on the surface of the body.

The endocrine system

The glands of the endocrine system produce over 50 different hormones, and most glands secrete more than one hormone. Hormones are also produced by individual cells or groups of cells in other tissues and organs. For example, the pancreatic islets, which produce the hormone insulin (it maintains the levels of blood sugar; see pp.137–139), are groups of cells that are found within the pancreas. The pancreas itself, however, is mostly an exocrine gland, releasing digestive hormones into a duct that connects to the duodenum, where the hormone can help digest food. Hormone-producing cells are also found in the walls of the small intestine, the stomach, the kidneys, the heart and the brain.

The endocrine system complements the nervous system. But whereas nerve impulses act quickly, hormones tend to act over a longer period of time – from 20 minutes to several hours, depending on the hormone. Some hormones exert their effects almost immediately, but others take hours, days or even years for their effects to become apparent. Adrenaline, for example, manufactured by the adrenal glands in reponse to stress, causes an almost instant speeding up of the heart. By contrast, the male hormone testosterone affects the development of the brain while the foetus is still in the uterus, but its effects may not be evident until many years after the child is born.

Changing roles

Each gland in the body has a specific job, but it also works in harmony with other glands. Some hormones are only active at certain times in a person's life, and their function can change with time. For example, growth hormone produced by the pituitary and thyroid glands control growth during childhood, but these same hormones have different roles in adults. The ovaries and testicles, or gonads, lie dormant in childhood and make hormones only when the child reaches puberty.

How hormones work

Hormones travel in the bloodstream to various tissues and organs, where they exert their influence. The major hormones circulate to virtually all the body's tissues, but each hormone acts on only certain cells, known as target cells. Each target cell has receptors on its surface, which allow it to respond to only a particular hormone. Receptors are molecules with a special shape, on to which the hormone binds, a bit like a key fitting into a lock. Once the hormone binds to a receptor, it is able to act within the target cell.

The levels of some hormones in the bloodstream are controlled by a complex biochemical cycle, known as a feedback loop (see right), which responds to the body's changing needs. The hypothalamus detects the levels of hormones in the blood. When they drop or increase beyond a normal level, the hypothalamus triggers the pituary gland to adjust its production of trophic hormone, which affects the amount of hormones other glands make. For example, when there is not enough thyroid hormone, more trophic hormone is produced; too much thyroid hormone, less trophic hormone is made. Factors that can affect hormone levels are food, exercise, age, illness and the time of the day or year.

SEE ALSO

Reaching puberty — **28–29**
Digestion — **90–91**
The brain and nervous system — **164–165**

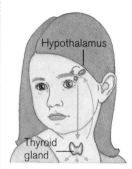

Normal hormone level

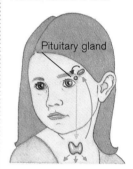

Too much thyroid hormone

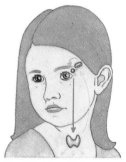

Too little thyroid hormone

The feedback loop

When the hypothalamus detects an increase or drop of a hormone, it prompts the pituitary to adjust its level of trophic hormone, which triggers the relevant gland to modify its hormone level.

Thyroid problems

The general rate of a child's growth, his metabolism and his sexual development are regulated by hormones that are produced by the thyroid gland. An underactive thyroid is present in about 1 in every 4,000 births.

A child's normal physical and mental development depends on the thryoid gland being able to maintain the appropriate levels of hormones. Hypothyroidism is the term used to describe an underactive thyroid that cannot produce enough hormones. In the past, when hypothyroidism sometimes went undiagnosed, children developed permanent brain damage and learning disabilities. This condition was known as cretinism, from which the word cretin derives.

In newborn babies, hypothyroidism may occur because the thyroid is absent, in the wrong position or not functioning properly, or because there is underactivity of the hypothalamus or pituitary gland, which is responsible for regulating the thyroid. It can also occur if a pregnant woman has an overactive thyroid and had to take antithyroid medication during pregnancy. Hypothyroidism may also be the result of an inherited disorder. In older children, hypothyroidism may be caused by thyroid disease or by underactivity of the hypothalamus or pituitary gland.

Treating hypothyroidism

All newborn babies are tested for hypothyroidism. If your baby has an underactive thyroid, he will be prescribed treatment with thyroxine, the main hormone produced by the thyroid gland. Babies identified and treated early will develop normally. In older children, the first sign of hypothyroidism may be goitre (opposite). Other signs include poor growth, lack of energy, poor appetite, increased weight gain, sensitivity to cold, pale, dry, itchy skin and constipation.

Blood tests will usually reveal low levels of thyroid hormones and raised levels of thyroid stimulating hormone (TSH), which is produced by the pituitary. Treatment is also with thyroxine. Once the child begins treatment, the symptoms will subside, although he will have to take thyroxine for the rest of his life.

Hyperthyroidism

Overactivity of the thyroid gland can result in hyperthyroidism. Neonatal hyperthyroidism affects newborn babies whose mothers have an overactive thyroid. It occurs when antibodies pass from the

The thyroid gland

A butterfly-shaped gland, the thyroid stretches across the front of the trachea, or windpipe. It produces several hormones, including thyroxine.

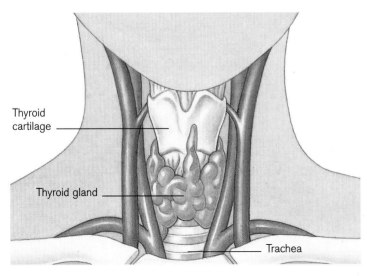

Thyroid cartilage

Thyroid gland

Trachea

mother's bloodstream to the unborn baby through the placenta.

Typical symptoms include prominent eyes, irritability, flushing of the skin and a fast pulse. In mild cases, the condition often disappears of its own accord without treatment once the antibodies pass out of the baby's bloodstream, usually within 3 to 12 weeks. Occasionally, symptoms may be more severe and the baby may be prescribed antithyroid drugs. These will be discontinued once the thyroid antibodies disappear.

In older children, hyperthyroidism can be difficult to diagnose. The child may have the typical symptoms of an overactive thyroid, such as goitre (see below), bulging eyes, hyperactivity, restlessness and a sudden increase in growth. A rapid pulse, increased nervousness, sweating and shakiness are other symptoms. Schoolwork may be affected and the child may become more easily upset than usual.

The doctor may take a blood sample to check the levels of thyroid hormones. If the levels are high, treatment with an antithyroid drug will usually bring the condition under control within a few weeks. In some cases, the condition disappears after a period of treatment. In others, the child has to continue treatment for the rest of his life. Occasionally, if treatment fails to control the condition, the doctor may suggest performing an operation to remove some of the thyroid gland surgically.

Goitre

An enlarged thyroid gland is known as goitre. It may appear at any age, but it is especially common in girls at the time they begin menstruating. In younger children, goitre may be caused by a mild inflammation of the thyroid gland, by a

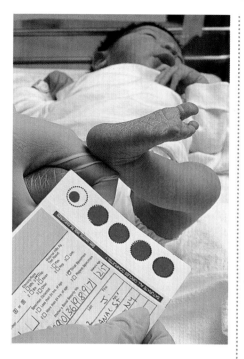

The Guthrie test

All newborns have a heel prick test, in which a small sample of blood is taken from the heel within a week of birth. It detects hypothyroidism, as well as the metabolic disorder known as phenylketonuria (PKU).

viral infection or by an underactive or overactive thyroid. The doctor may perform tests to determine if the goitre is caused by a problem that requires treatment. In developing countries, goitre can be caused by too little iodine in the diet, which is added to table salt in industrialized countries.

SWOLLEN GLANDS

What we erroneously refer to as swollen glands are, in fact, enlarged lymph nodes (known medically as lymphadenopathy). They are usually caused by a minor viral or bacterial infection. The swelling is a result of the accumulation of white blood cells – the lymphocytes – which are produced by the immune system to fight the infection. Swollen glands are especially common in children, perhaps because the lymphatic system plays a greater role in fighting off infection during childhood. Occasionally, swollen glands may be caused by an allergic reaction. More rarely, they may be a sign of a serious illness such as leukaemia or Hodgkin's disease.

Swollen glands may be felt as tender, slightly warm lumps about the size of a pea. They commonly occur in the neck, armpits and groin, and those that swell tend to be the ones nearest to the site of the infection. For example, swollen glands in the neck are often associated with a throat infection.

Growth hormone deficiency

When the pituitary gland fails to make enough of the growth hormone somatotropin – this occurs in 1 in every 4,000 children – a child can fail to grow at a normal rate.

Measuring up

Routine health checks may show that a child is growing more slowly than normal, a sign of a growth disorder.

The problem may be noticed during routine health checks or if your child is short and looks young for her age. One sign of the deficiency is that the child is obese, despite eating normally – the growth hormone helps control the amount of fatty tissue under the skin.

Growth hormone deficiency may be caused by a problem in the hypothalamus, with the link between the hypothalamus and the pituitary gland or with the pituitary itself. Sometimes it is linked to deficiencies of other hormones. The condition may be inherited – about 3 percent of children with it have a sibling who has it too. In other cases, the pituitary gland is underdeveloped or absent, or has been damaged during birth or by a head injury. Pituitary failure can also be a result of a pituitary or brain tumour or treatment for leukaemia (see p.117). However, in the vast majority of cases, no cause can be identified.

Some children are short in stature, even though they have no shortage of growth hormone. They often come from families where one or both parents are short.

Diagnosis and treatment

Your doctor can use blood tests to check if a hormone deficiency is the problem. If it is, the child may be prescribed synthetic growth hormone, which must be injected every day, usually just before bedtime. Devices are available, which are also used to treat diabetes, to make injections more tolerable. The child's growth will be measured at regular intervals to assess her response to treatment. Because growth hormone deficient children can become obese, it is vital to encourage your child to eat a well-balanced, nutritious diet (see p.34) and to be active. The specialist can refer her to a dietitian.

Treatment stops when the child reaches adulthood. There is a good chance that she will attain a reasonable height. Her final height depends on the age at which she was diagnosed and treatment began, which should be by the age of six.

OTHER GROWTH DISORDERS

Growth disorders can be a result of other disorders, such as cystic fibrosis (see p.148), coeliac disease (see pp.98–99) or renal or cardiac problems. It can also occur because of chromosomal abnormalities. Turner's syndrome is the most common one, affecting 1 in every 2,500 girls. It is caused by a lack or partial lack of one of the X chromosomes. The girl is short and may have puffy hands and feet, webbing of the neck, a broad chest, small nipples and a characteristic face. A girl with the disorder rarely attains more than 147 cm (4 ft 10 in) in height as an adult. Her growth hormone secretion is almost always normal; however, it has been found that giving her synthetic growth hormone can dramatically increase her growth, but it is not known how this will affect her final adult height.

Gigantism – excessive tallness – may be the result of having tall parents or it may be caused by overproduction of a growth hormone. This may be the result of a pituitary tumour or of overproduction of a releasing hormone or underproduction of somatostatin, which controls growth hormone secretion by the hypothalamus. Diagnosis is made using a brain scan and blood tests, and treatment may involve a drug that blocks the release of growth hormone or surgery.

Diabetes

One of the most common chronic diseases is diabetes – or diabetes mellitus, to use the correct medical term. The disease occurs in 1 in every 500 children, when the body does not make enough insulin.

Insulin is a hormone manufactured by the pancreas, and it enables cells to produce and use glucose, the body's main source of energy. Glucose is a simple sugar, produced by the digestion of carbohydrate or starchy foods. In normal circumstances, immediately after eating a meal, the pancreas secretes insulin, which allows the body's tissues to absorb glucose from the food and prevents blood glucose levels from rising too high. Between meals, the level of insulin in the bloodstream falls. The body then draws glucose from stores in the liver to prevent glucose levels from dropping too low.

In diabetics, the pancreas either does not make any insulin at all or does not produce enough, or the cells of the body do not respond normally to it. As a result, the levels of glucose in the blood rise. The body tries to rid itself of this excess glucose, causing the typical symptoms of diabetes (see p.138). If untreated, diabetes can lead to coma and death. Once treated with insulin, symptoms rapidly improve and, with good medical management, the person can lead a normal life.

Insulin-dependent diabetes

The type of diabetes that affects children is known as type 1, or insulin-dependent diabetes mellitus (IDDM), formerly known as juvenile diabetes. (Non-insulin dependent diabetes, or type 2 diabetes, mainly affects adults, especially those who are overweight.)

Insulin-dependent diabetes mellitus can occur at any time in childhood. It is an autoimmune disease that occurs when the body's immune system mistakenly destroys the pancreatic cells, which produce insulin. The disorder runs in families, so if you or your partner has IDDM, your child has a 5 percent chance of developing it, but other environmental factors are needed before the child develops the disease.

In the case of IDDM, it is not known what causes the body to turn against itself. One theory is that a virus mimics normal proteins in the pancreas in an attempt to evade the body's immune response. This, in turn, causes the immune system to become sensitized to its own cells and it attacks the pancreas, leading to a loss of the insulin-producing cells.

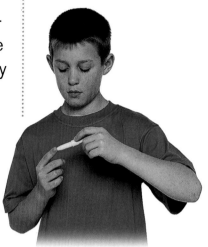

Testing glucose levels
A finger-pricking device is necessary to provide a drop of blood to test glucose levels. Automatic devices are available that prick the skin fast and with minimum discomfort.

DIABETES INSIPIDUS

The rare condition diabetes insipidus, in which a child is excessively thirsty and passes large amounts of urine, has nothing to do with insulin deficiency. It occurs when the pituitary gland fails to secrete antidiuretic hormone (ADH), which reduces the amount of water passed by the kidneys into the urine. It may be caused by a congenital defect, kidney disease or destruction or damage to the tissues of the hypothalamus or pituitary. A form of the disorder, nephrogenic diabetes insipidus, is caused by a defect in the urinary concentration mechanism in the kidneys.

Diagnosis is by means of urine analysis and other tests. If the pituitary gland is failing to produce ADH, treatment involves giving ADH replacement therapy. However, this is not effective in the nephrogenic form, which normally is treated by a low-sodium diet and diuretic drugs.

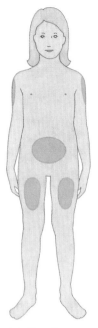

The injection sites

Injecting insulin in the same site can cause scarring, so injections are rotated among the fatty areas of the body: the upper arms, the abdomen and the thighs.

Establishing a routine

The number of insulin injections needed varies. Most children require two injections a day: one before breakfast and one before their evening meal.

Early symptoms

IDDM develops quickly, often over a few weeks. The body attempts to rid itself of extra glucose by excreting it in the urine, causing frequent urination. You may notice bed-wetting after the child has previously been dry or frequent trips to the lavatory. This leads to increased thirst and drinking. In girls, glucose in the urine may contribute to vaginal thrush. Because insulin helps build muscles and increases stores of fat, a shortage of insulin will lead to a break down of muscle and, even though the child is eating enough food, she will begin to lose weight.

In older children, these symptoms are obvious. However, diabetes can be hard to diagnose in younger children. If she is still in nappies, increased urination is masked, and crying because of thirst may be misinterpreted. Weight loss may also be difficult to spot because younger children do not have a lot of body fat and are often faddy eaters.

Diagnosis involves testing the child's urine for glucose. Blood tests will also be performed to check glucose levels in the

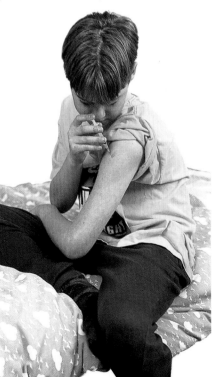

blood. If your child is diagnosed with diabetes, she will be referred to a specialist childhood diabetes clinic at the hospital, where she will have access to an experienced team of experts.

Insulin treatment

The three mainstays of treatment are insulin, diet and exercise. The aim is to control your child's glucose levels in order to ensure that she grows and develops normally. With good control, there is every likelihood that your child will grow up healthy and avoid potential long-term complications caused by high blood glucose levels such as damage to the eyes, kidneys, heart and nervous system.

Because insulin would be digested in the stomach if taken orally, it must be injected. Insulin comes in two types. The first is a clear short-acting insulin that lasts about six to eight hours, with a peak action at three to four hours. The intermediate or slow-acting type is opaque and looks thick. Once injected, it begins to act after 1 to 2 hours and its effects last for up to 14 hours. The type of insulin and the number of injections prescribed for your child will be tailored to her individual needs. Insulin may be injected with a syringe or a pen-needle device that contains a cartridge of insulin.

Treating hypoglycaemia

Too little glucose in the blood is known as hypoglycaemia. It may be caused by too much insulin, missing a meal or a sudden bout of exercise. The child may tremble, sweat, feel dizzy or be confused or have abdominal pain. Left untreated, hypoglycaemia can lead to seizures and unconsciousness. The child should immediately eat or drink something sweet, such as a biscuit, chocolate or a sweet drink (but not those labelled "diet".

or "lite", which may not have sugar), to boost her levels of blood sugar. If your child refuses to eat or drink or if her blood glucose level falls so low that she becomes drowsy or loses consciousness, you need to give an injection of glucagon (a hormone that causes the liver to release glucose into the bloodstream) to bring the glucose level back to normal. If the hypoglycaemia becomes advanced, call the doctor or take your child to the nearest accident and emergency department.

Testing glucose levels

Regular testing of glucose levels is necessary to ensure that the child is receiving the correct amount of insulin. This involves pricking the finger with a special lancet to obtain a drop of blood. The blood is dropped on to a testing strip, which reacts chemically with the glucose. One type of strip changes colour and can be compared with a colour chart to give the blood glucose level. The other type of strip is inserted into a portable monitoring device to provide a more precise blood glucose reading.

Diet and exercise

The current recommendation is that the most appropriate dietary regime is the same as that recommended for health for everyone – that is, a balanced combination of foods based around fruit, vegetables and wholegrain cereals, with a small amount of protein and occasional fatty and sugary foods, spread over three meals and two snacks a day. Diabetic control is better if meals and snacks are taken at the same times each day to prevent low blood glucose levels if meals are skipped or delayed and to avoid high blood glucose levels if meals are eaten too close together.

Although life-saving, treatment for diabetes is not always easy, and your child will need a good deal of encouragement from you and the medical team treating her diabetes, especially in the early days. With good management, your child should be able to live a normal, active life and grow up strong and healthy, although she will have to have daily insulin injections for the rest of her life. Most children get used to injecting themselves and testing their blood glucose levels.

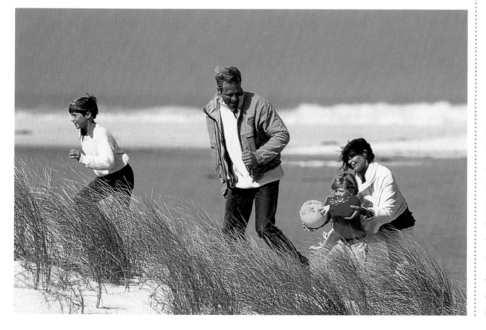

Keeping active

If your child has diabetes, he should be encouraged to participate in regular exercise, sports and family outings. If travelling across time zones, seek medical advise to adjust her insulin schedule.

Genetic disorders

The colour of a child's eyes and hair are only two of the characteristics determined by his genes, which are inherited from his parents. The genes determine other factors, including mental and physical disorders.

The basic genetic building blocks are genes, which are formed from DNA, the substance in cells that provides the blueprint for growth in every living organism. Genes are grouped together as chromosomes. There are 46 chromosomes in each cell, divided into 23 pairs. The only cells that don't have 46 chromosomes are the egg and the sperm. They have 23 each, so a child receives half his genes from his mother and half from his father. Any genetic abnormality must have been present in either the egg or the sperm or in both.

Genetic disorders occur when the DNA sends out a wrong message. They are inherited in different ways, depending on whether the defective gene is dominant or recessive. When the gene is dominant, the baby needs to receive the defective gene from only one parent to have the condition; when it is recessive, both parents must be carriers. There is also a gender-linked route – or x-linked inheritance – in which the mother is a carrier and unaffected but may pass on a serious genetic abnormality to her sons. Her daughters will not be affected but run a 50 percent chance of being carriers of the disease.

Many embryos with genetic disorders do not survive – they are usually lost within the first few months of pregnancy through miscarriage. When the pregnancy does continue, there are a number of tests (see box, opposite) that can be carried out to check for abnormalities.

A blood sample is used to inspect the chromosomes for any problems. The cells are broken open, and the chromosomes

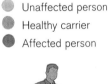

- Unaffected person
- Healthy carrier
- Affected person

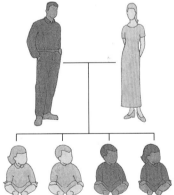

Dominant inheritance

A defective gene from only one parent has a one in two chance of being passed on to a child.

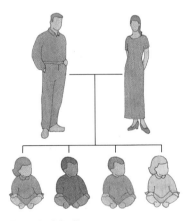

Recessive inheritance

If both parents are carriers, the chances of a child being a carrier is one in two and of getting the disease is one in four.

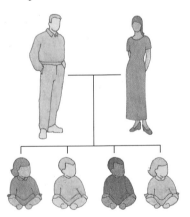

X-linked inheritance

A female carrier has a one in two chance of passing on the disease to a son or making a daughter a carrier.

are dyed and put under a microscope so that the pairs can be counted. Any deviation from the 23 pairs means that there is a genetic abnormality, the most common one being Down's syndrome. More sophisticated tests can reveal some chromosome problems that do not cause a change in the number of chromosomes.

When to be tested

A woman should be offered testing during pregnancy (see box, below) if she or her partner has an affected family member, if she has already given birth to an affected baby or if she falls into another high-risk group.

For many parents, having prior knowledge that their baby is likely to be born with a genetic defect is a positive advantage that past generations did not have. It gives them the power to make choices. They may decide to terminate the pregnancy, or they may decide to proceed with it – they will then have time to prepare and inform themselves about the disorder as much as possible before the baby is born. Parents who are at risk of giving birth to a child with a genetic abnormality, or already have a child with such a condition, may be able to have a healthy child through in vitro fertilization – the embryo can be checked for defects before being implanted in the womb.

Diagnosing a baby

Genetic abnormalities are not always identified in pregnancy, and it may be weeks, months or even years after birth before it becomes apparent that something is wrong, depending upon the nature of the disease. Down's syndrome and phenylketonuria are two conditions that can be diagnosed early after birth through blood tests. Other conditions,

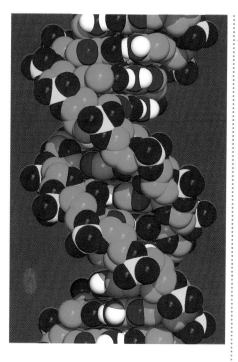

SEE ALSO

Down's syndrome	142–143
Leukaemia	117
Phenylketonuria	147
Cystic fibrosis	148

The DNA molecule
Your genes are made of DNA, which controls growth and all the body's functions. The model here is colour-coded to indicate the atoms that make up DNA: oxygen (red), carbon (green), nitrogen (blue), hydrogen (white) and phosphorus (yellow).

such as sickle cell anaemia and cystic fibrosis, may only become apparent when the baby is a few months old or even older, when the symptoms begin to appear. A diagnosis of a genetic disorder can be confirmed by testing for the symptoms caused by the abnormal gene or by trying to find the abnormal chromosome or gene itself.

TESTING DURING PREGNANCY

There are two types of tests taken during pregnancy: screening tests and diagnostic tests. Those that screen are only able to tell a woman if she is at risk of having a baby with a genetic disorder but are not conclusive. For example, the blood tests for Down's syndrome identify some babies as being at risk who don't have the condition, yet miss others who are born with the disorder.

Older women or those who have a high risk will be offered diagnostic tests, which should show for certain if the baby has a particular condition. Chorionic villus sampling and amniocentesis are diagnostic tests (see p.144). They are not 100 percent accurate but mistakes are rarely made, especially with amniocentesis, which is carried out later in the pregnancy; both carry a risk of miscarriage. An ultrasound scan can be classified as both a screening and diagnostic test, depending on the nature of the disorder.

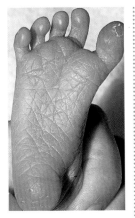

Skin creases

The soles of the feet and the palms of the hands of children with Down's syndrome are characterized by abnormal skin creases.

Down's syndrome

One of the most common congenital disorders is Down's syndrome, in which a combination of symptoms affects a child. One baby in about 700 is born with the syndrome, which occurs in all ethnic groups.

The syndrome is caused by a defect in the chromosomes and is present from the moment of conception. The foetus has an extra chromosome – 47 instead of 46. A diagnosis of Down's syndrome is often made at birth because of the characteristic features of a child with this disorder (see chart, opposite). However, the condition is not always obvious in the early hours after birth, and a diagnosis can only be certain after a chromosome test.

Many children with Down's syndrome will live a healthy life, but there are some medical problems that are more common in Down's children. For example, about 40 percent of babies have a heart problem at birth (see pp.118–119), which may need surgery, and up to 30 percent of those with Down's develop a thyroid disorder. More than 50 percent of Down's children have a hearing problem, and vision problems

are more prevalent. They are also more prone to chest infections such as colds.

The average growth of children with Down's syndrome is different from that of the rest of the population. They tend to be shorter and put on weight more readily. Special charts are available to monitor the growth of a Down's child.

Treatment and education

Caring for a baby with Down's syndrome involves some extra steps. In the first two weeks it may be difficult for the baby to suck and swallow milk. If you want to breastfeed, you may have to keep your milk going until your baby can cope. Because the thyroid may not function

Learning for the future

A Down's syndrome child is unlikely to be totally self-sufficient, but many can learn and lead relatively normal lives; as adults, some manage to hold down permanent jobs.

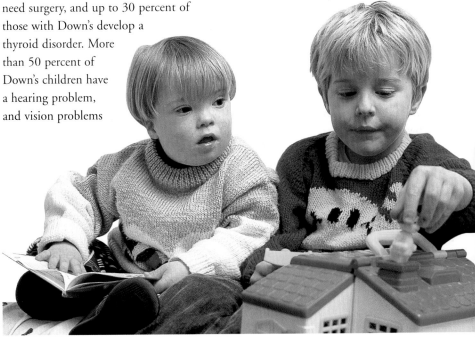

properly, the baby's mechanism to control her body heat may not work properly. It is important that she's not cold, but avoid overheating her (see pp.18–19). If your baby's skin is dry, massage it with some baby oil, moisturizing cream or olive oil. Playing games, such as pulling faces and making noises, will help your baby to improve control of her tongue.

The degree of learning disability varies enormously, but parents often discover that their child's potential far exceeds their expectations. In general, Down's children reach development stages later than the average child (for example, they exhibit the classic difficult behaviour of two year olds at four years of age), but they go on to make progress throughout their lives.

Despite a high incidence of hearing, sight and speech impairments, many Down's children are successfully educated in mainstream schools – certainly at nursery and primary levels, and some in secondary schools, where they have achieved good academic results.

Quality of life

Life expectancy has risen rapidly. In the past, people with this condition rarely survived beyond 30 years of age, but many now live to late middle age and beyond. This is due to the improved treatment of the conditions that often afflict people with Down's syndrome, including heart disease and severe chest infections. However, there is a higher risk of developing Alzheimer's disease (presenile dementia).

One important factor for Down's children is how they are perceived by society. Because of their appearance, they are easily identifiable, and many people make assumptions about their capabilities without giving them the chance to show what they can do. As with any group,

there are diverse levels of abilities and personality traits among Down's children.

Cosmetic surgery can change the appearance of a Down's child. Some parents have chosen it to help their child to integrate into society. There is debate on whether this surgery is ethical. One procedure removes part of the tongue to prevent it from protruding; another inserts silicone implants to change the shape of the nose, cheek and chin. These are major procedures and, if considered, should only be done after puberty.

SEE ALSO
Milestones	**22–27**
Genetic disorders	**140–141**
Hearing difficulties	**202–203**
Visual problems	**204–205**

HOW DOWN'S AFFECTS A CHILD

Differences	Symptoms
Characteristic features	• The outer corners of the eyes slant upward, and the inside corners are covered with folds of skin that extend from the bridge of the nose. • The face and its features are smaller than those of other children. • The tongue is enlarged and tends to protrude from the mouth, which makes eating and speech difficult. • The back of the head is flattened. • Both the hands and feet have abnormal skin creases. • The hands are broad and short, and the little fingers curve inward.
Physical disorders	• The ears are susceptible to infections; there may be congenital deafness. • One Down's child out of three suffers from a heart defect; it may need no treatment or may require surgery. • The lungs may be susceptible to infections. • Part of the intestine may be narrowed. • The thyroid may not produce enough hormone, causing slow growth and excessive weight gain. • There is developmental delay. • The ligaments in the neck may be weak, which can – rarely – lead to a serious spinal injury.

Fragile X syndrome

The genetically inherited disease known as fragile X syndrome can have serious implications for those affected by it. On average, 1 in 2,000 boys and 1 in 4,000 girls are born with the disease.

This syndrome occurs when a child inherits a fragile X chromosome from a parent. The affected child is usually a boy who inherits the abnormal chromosome from his mother. As he has only one X chromosome, the abnormality will become apparent. If a girl inherits the abnormal X chromosome, it will often be counterbalanced by a normal one, and the abnormality may be mild or may not exist

The outcome of fragile X syndrome for affected children is a learning disability, the intensity of which varies considerably from child to child. Boys are far more likely to suffer severe learning disabilities than girls; in fact only 30 to 40 percent of girls with this genetic inheritance will experience any learning difficulties at all.

Fragile X chromosome

The chromosome can be detected by DAPI staining (right) or FISH, which uses a fluorescent probe (far right). Arrows indicate the weak points.

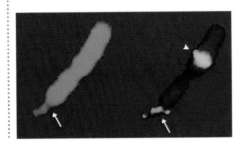

HOW FRAGILE X SYNDROME MANIFESTS

Children with fragile X often have delayed speech development, and as they get older other developmental delays may manifest themselves. The fingers of these children frequently have loose connective tissue and can be easily extended backward. The skin is usually thin and fine and facial features can be long and thin. Boys with fragile X may have large ears and a prominent forehead; they may also show signs of hyperactivity, repetitive behaviour and autism.

Genetic counselling

If you, your partner or any other family member is known to have fragile X and you are planning a pregnancy, or are pregnant already, you will be advised to see a genetic counsellor. The role of these counsellors is to inform you about the chances of the disease being inherited by your baby or any babies you may have in the future.

The counsellor will need a full medical history from you and your partner. If you are a female carrier – because you have one normal and one abnormal gene – there is a 50 percent chance that, if you have a son, he will inherit the disease. If you give birth to a daughter, there is a 50 percent chance she will be a carrier. If you have a brother with fragile X, you are probably a carrier.

Tests can be taken during pregnancy to identify if the problem chromosome is present. Chorionic villus sampling involves removing a tiny piece of placenta for chromosomal or biochemical testing. This takes place during the 10th week of pregnancy. Amniocentesis, which involves inserting a needle into the womb to remove a small amount of fluid with foetal cells, can be done at 16 weeks.

How you decide to act upon the results will depend upon your personal beliefs. If you are anti-abortion, you may prefer not to be tested; however, knowing the results of these tests will allow you to plan and gain more support, should you need it.

Thalassaemia

A type of anaemia, thalassaemia occurs when there is defective production of haemoglobin – the vital pigment in blood that is responsible for transporting oxygen around the body.

SEE ALSO

Heart, blood and
circulation   **114–115**
Bones, muscles
and joints   **120–121**

This genetically transmitted disorder is generally restricted to people of Asian and Mediterranean origin. The degree of severity of thalassaemia will depend on whether the child has inherited from his parents one or two abnormal genes (see pp.140–141). If there is only one thalassaemia gene present, the child will usually have no symptoms – however, women with this problem may become anaemic during pregnancy. This condition is often referred to as thalassaemia minor.

Thalassaemia genes inherited from both parents will leave the child unable to produce any haemoglobin, apart from that which is made in the womb and in early infancy. This condition is potentially fatal, but it can be alleviated through treatment. This form of the disease is often called thalassaemia major or, sometimes, Cooley's anaemia.

If a baby is suffering from the severe form of thalassaemia, he will become chronically anaemic during his first 12 months and will suffer from breathlessness and have difficulty feeding properly. The red blood cells break up rapidly, causing an enlarged liver and spleen, which means that the baby's abdomen will appear distended.

If left untreated, the bone marrow will begin to expand, which can eventually lead to unusual bone growth and an enlarged skull. Body growth will stop and the child will die in early childhood.

THE KEY TO TREATMENT

A child with thalassaemia can be successfully treated, but the condition must be identified quickly so that blood transfusions can be given every three to four weeks; these continue for life.

Regular transfusions will cause an accumulation of iron, so injections of a drug to prevent excess iron build-up will be necessary. In some cases, the spleen may need to be removed. A future cure may come in the form of a bone marrow transplant.

Thalassaemia can be diagnosed by examining a sample of the child's blood under a microscope. If you or your partner have relatives with thalassaemia, you should consider genetic counselling before trying to conceive children.

Telltale signs

Symptoms usually appear when a baby is three to six months old. They include fatigue and shortness of breath.

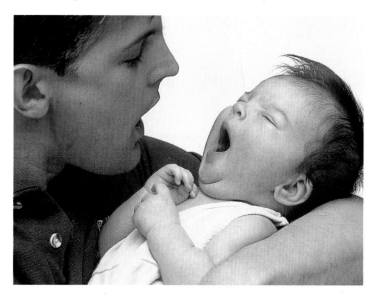

Haemophilia

Normally, blood contains clotting factors that are needed to stop bleeding. In haemophilia, a genetically inherited disease, one of the clotting factors is missing or there is a shortage of it, which leads to excessive bleeding.

Taking exercise

A haemophiliac doesn't have to avoid all sports, only those with physical contact. Swimming and walking are ideal choices.

There are two forms of this disorder – classical haemophilia (haemophilia A) and Christmas disease (haemophilia B). Both types produce the same symptoms.

The gene for haemophilia is carried by females, who do not have the disease, but

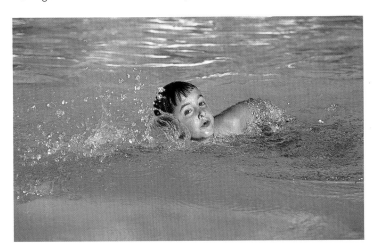

there is a 50 percent chance of a son being affected and a 50 percent chance of a daughter being a carrier. A haemophiliac cannot pass the disease on to his son but any daughters will be carriers.

You should obtain genetic counselling if this disease affects your family. To prepare yourself, you can have amniocentesis to detect the sex of your unborn child. The test, performed in the 16th week of pregnancy, involves inserting a needle into the abdomen to collect some amniotic fluid, which can then be analysed.

When treatment is necessary

The symptoms vary considerably because the affected clotting factor in the blood may be present in reduced amounts or may be completely absent. If the child is missing a clotting factor completely, there will be incidents of spontaneous, painful bleeding into the joints and muscles and, if he suffers a large cut, bleeding will be intense and he may need hospitalization. Boys who have some of the clotting factor may not have spontaneous bleeding, but accidents and operations will cause excessive bleeding.

It was once impossible to prevent bleeding into the joints and muscles, which can cause debilitating physical deformities. Currently, the disease is treated with injections of the missing clotting factor. If the haemophilia is severe, injections are needed whenever bleeding occurs; but in less seriously affected boys, treatment is needed only prior to an operation or dental extraction.

You should be able to trust an older child to know when symptoms call for treatment, but closely watch a young child to prevent accidents and, if one occurs, to get treatment as soon as possible.

HAEMOPHILIA AND AIDS

The missing factors that haemophiliacs need are obtained from donor blood, and some haemophiliacs contracted the HIV virus before the implications of AIDS became apparent. Now, however, all blood donors are carefully screened and all blood that is used is treated to minimize any risk. Synthetic clotting factors are also becoming available, and these will negate any risk of infection.

Phenylketonuria

An enzyme deficiency can cause phenylketonuria, or PKU – a rare, but serious, inherited metabolic disorder. It is estimated that the disease affects about 1 in every 15,000 newborn babies.

SEE ALSO

Thyroid problems   134–135
Genetic disorders   140–141
Identifying a child with developmental delay   196–197

Normally, the body produces an enzyme to convert phenylalanine, an amino acid present in food, into the amino acid tyrosine. If this process cannot take place, it results in too much phenylalanine being present in the body.

A newborn baby with the condition is not affected; however, if it is left untreated, by early infancy the child will develop neurological problems, including epilepsy, seizures and learning difficulties. The child will have a musty smell due to the high levels of phenylalanine in his urine and he may develop eczema (see pp.102–103).

There is a simple test available to determine whether or not the disorder is present. The Guthrie, or heel prick test, is usually carried out when the baby is between 5 and 14 days old and consists of a small prick to the heel. The blood from the prick is gathered on special blotting paper and tested for a few serious conditions, including PKU.

To reduce the discomfort associated with the test, place an extra pair of socks or booties on his feet before the test is carried out; this will ensure that his feet are warm and make the test less painful. Feed your child immediately after the test and any discomfort will soon be soothed away.

Living with PKU

If phenylketonuria is discovered, you will be advised on how to give your child a diet low in phenylalanine. This will mean that he can eat only foods low in protein. It can be difficult to keep your child restricted to a low-protein diet, but it will prevent the mental disabilities that can occur if he doesn't follow it.

Regular blood tests will be taken to monitor your child's condition. It was once thought that an adult with the disorder can have a normal diet, but research indicates that a diet low in phenylalanine should be continued for life.

THE PKU DIET

A baby with PKU should have a small amount of a special formula that is low in phenylalanine, followed by breast milk, or a small amount of normal baby formula, followed by the special formula.

Solid foods for weaning can be introduced at four to six months; follow advice from the dietitian. In general, all fruit can be given, as can most vegetables and some baby foods. High-protein foods such as meats, dairy products, eggs and pasta and grains must be avoided. The diet will eventually include low-protein foods, but some of these will only be available on prescription, including special breads, pasta and biscuits.

Balancing act
Your child will have to carefully monitor the food she eats, but she can enjoy some of the snack foods all children love.

Cystic fibrosis

The most commonly inherited disease among European people is cystic fibrosis – it is rarely found in Afro-Caribbean or Asian people. As many as 1 in every 25 Caucasian people is a carrier of the disease.

In order for cystic fibrosis to manifest, both parents must be carriers. Most carriers have no symptoms of the disease, but if there is a family history of cystic fibrosis, a test can be taken to determine if you and your partner are carriers. This involves providing a mouth wash sample. The test is not 100 percent accurate and parents can only know for certain whether their unborn child has the disease after chorionic villus sampling or amniocentesis.

Cystic fibrosis may be detected in the first few days after birth if there is a build-up of the waste products the baby usually passes soon after birth. It can lead to a bowel obstruction, but only a minority of babies suffer this early complication. Sometimes the condition isn't detected for months, even years, after the child has suffered much ill health.

Living with cystic fibrosis

A child with cystic fibrosis produces a sticky mucus that builds up in the lungs and respiratory passages, the nose and the sinuses. From an early age, it causes severe and frequent respiratory infections, and often the lungs become damaged if treatment doesn't begin early on. The child will also have digestive problems because the pancreas fails to secrete sufficient enzymes to break down fats. Weight gain will be slow and anaemia is common.

Despite the severity of the condition, the quality of life for a child with cystic fibrosis has improved considerably because newer medications have become increasingly effective in fighting lung infection and pancreatic problems. The child is usually able to live a fairly normal life and take part in most of the same activities as her friends, provided she follows a strict regime of physiotherapy and medication.

A highly nutritious diet is also essential if the child is to maintain a normal weight, and school meals should be monitored carefully to make sure she is getting enough calories. The sweat glands are also affected by the condition and excrete excessive amounts of salt, so the child should have extra salt. This is particularly important in hot weather.

In extreme cases, heart and lung transplants may be necessary, but they are proving successful.

Daily routine

Carers are trained to carry out intensive physiotherapy three times a day, which enables the child to cough up some of the sticky mucus that builds up in his lungs.

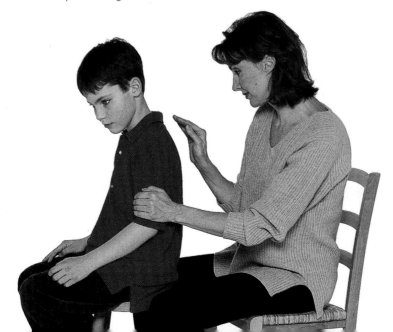

Sickle cell anaemia

It is mainly people of Afro-Caribbean origin and sometimes those of Asian or Middle Eastern origin who are affected by the disorder known as sickle cell anaemia, so called because of the abnormal shape of the red blood cells.

SEE ALSO

Caring for your child
in hospital   **56–57**

Heart, blood and
circulation   **114–115**

This blood disorder occurs when there is an abnormality in the structure of haemoglobin – the substance in the red blood cells that carries oxygen – and the red blood cells cannot form into the typical spherical shape. It has been shown that sickle-shaped cells offer protection against malaria, which is why it mainly affects people from countries where malaria is common.

It takes two sickle cell genes to cause the disease (see pp.140–141). If both parents are carriers of the condition – they have the gene but not the disease – there is a 25 percent chance that a child will have the disease, a 50 percent chance that a child will be a carrier and a 25 percent chance that a child will neither have the disease nor be a carrier. If one parent has the disease but the other parent doesn't and isn't a carrier, the children may be carriers but won't have the disease.

How it affects the child

A blood test from both the child and the parents will be taken to confirm the diagnosis. Children with sickle cell anaemia are usually diagnosed at about the age of six months, when swellings on their hands and feet become noticeable. The abnormal red blood cells form into clumps and attack growing bones. When the bone becomes damaged, new bone will grow over it, causing the swellings. The disease also affects the spleen, which becomes enlarged and painful.

As the child grows she will probably suffer increasing bouts of pain – known as crises – in which the misformed red blood cells cause the blood supply to an organ to be reduced or cut off altogether. They often occur after she has become dehydrated as a result of an infection, and they are usually accompanied by fever. Any part of the body can be affected – the kidneys, liver, lungs or even the brain.

Children with the condition now live into adulthood. Prompt medication, such as painkillers and antibiotic drugs, and oxygen therapy will help a child to cope during a crisis, and a blood transfusion may be necessary. At present the only cure for sickle cell anaemia is a bone marrow transplant, but this is rarely performed.

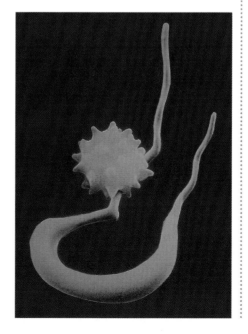

Red blood cells

Normal red blood cells are spherical in shape; those of a person with sickle cell anaemia have an elongated, curved shape and are rigid.

The mouth and teeth

Strong, healthy teeth are vital for chewing food, and a bright smile will help your child look and feel confident. Establishing dental care habits from an early age will ensure your child has healthy teeth and gums.

A simple routine of daily brushing, combined with a balanced diet and regular visits to the dentist or hygienist, will ensure that your child has healthy teeth and gums and stays free from dental and oral problems.

Brushing and flossing

From the ages of two to about eight you should help your child to brush his teeth twice a day. Unless you live in an area where the water is fluoridated, it is recommended that your child use a toothpaste containing 1,000–1,500 ppm of fluoride to help form strong teeth, because low-fluoride formulations are less effective in helping to prevent tooth decay. A fluoride supplement is also available. Rinsing with water immediately after brushing with a fluoride toothpaste will reduce its effectiveness, so encourage your child simply to spit out the paste.

Although fluoride makes tooth enamel resistant to attack from plaque, too much fluoride may cause the teeth to become mottled. You should check fluoride levels in your water supply and ask your dentist if more fluoride is needed before giving your child a supplement.

When choosing a toothbrush for your child, look for one with a small head; compact, soft to medium filaments; and a wide handle, which makes the brush easier for him to manipulate. The filaments should be nylon, with rounded ends, to avoid damaging the soft tissues of the mouth. Choose an attractive, brightly coloured toothbrush to help maintain your child's interest in brushing.

A young child will often want to use a toothbrush by himself, but he may not be very efficient at brushing his teeth. Always supervise him and be prepared to finish the task. As your child get older, he

Brushing teeth

As your child gets older, you should encourage her to brush and floss her teeth on her own.

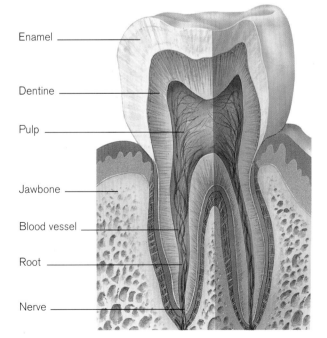

Enamel

Dentine

Pulp

Jawbone

Blood vessel

Root

Nerve

Anatomy of the tooth

The outer surface of each tooth visible above the gum line is enamel, the hardest substance in the human body. Beneath this, another hard layer, dentine, encloses the pulp – soft tissue rich in blood vessels and nerve endings. The tooth roots fit into a socket in the jawbone.

can take over more of his own oral hygiene routine. It is less essential for a child to floss than it is for an adult; however, by establishing the habit at an early age, flossing will become part of your child's normal oral hygiene routine. The dentist or hygienist can show him the best way to do it.

Tooth decay

Brushing teeth helps prevent tooth decay, or dental caries. They start with plaque, the thin, sticky film that forms on the teeth. Bacteria in plaque, such as *Lactobacillus acidophilus* and *Streptococcus mutans*, metabolize sugars found in food into acids that attack the tooth enamel. Because plaque is sticky, the acids are kept in contact with the tooth enamel, which can cause demineralization – a loss of calcium and phosphate.

Over time, the tooth enamel and underlying dentine are broken down, and decay attacks the pulp at the centre of the tooth. This may become infected, which can lead to permanent damage to nerves and blood vessels. If your child complains of toothache, the hard enamel of the tooth has already been eroded.

Visiting the dentist

At a check up, the dentist will examine your child's teeth, and he may take X-rays. If there are early signs of decay, the dentist may clean the teeth and scrape them to remove plaque. This enables saliva to remineralize the enamel.

If tooth decay has progressed further, the dentist may have to remove the decay, using a drill, and replace it with a filling. If decay has reached the pulp, infection and death of the pulp is inevitable and the pulp may have to be removed and the root canal filled. If the decay is more advanced, the tooth may be extracted.

Positioning of the teeth

A poor fit between the upper and lower teeth when they bite together is known as malocclusion. Sometimes the teeth are so crowded and crooked that they look unattractive. Malocclusion can also put a strain on the jaw muscles and make the teeth difficult to clean, increasing the risk of tooth decay and gum, jaw and joint problems. Orthodontic treatment, which may involve removing some teeth and fitting braces, can correct overcrowding and misalignment. Treatment usually begins from about the age of 11, but age is less important than the presence of the correct number of teeth.

SEE ALSO

Healthy family eating	**34**
Teeth and tooth care	**38–39**
Mouth-related problems	**152–153**

DIFFERENT TYPES OF BRACES

Orthodontic appliances work by applying gentle, sustained pressure to the teeth, causing them to move into a new position. As they move, the bone beneath the teeth is remodelled so that the teeth remain in position. The appliances may be fixed or removable and may have to be worn for anything from a few months to two and a half years or more. The child will have to visit an orthodontist at four to six week intervals for adjustments as the teeth shift position.

When only a few teeth need correcting, removable appliances are normally used. The brace is fixed to a plate that covers the roof of the mouth and can be taken out for cleaning. The brace has delicate wires and springs that gradually move the teeth by exerting gentle pressure.

Fixed braces have brackets and bands that are temporarily stuck to the teeth so they cannot be removed. A flexible wire joins the brackets, allowing the teeth to be moved. Fixed braces are usually made of metal, but plastic and ceramic appliances, which are less obvious, are also available.

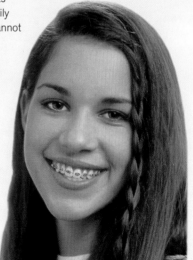

In addition to fixed or removable appliances, headgear may be needed to apply extra pressure to specific teeth. It usually needs to be worn only in the evening or at night.

Mouth-related problems

Children sometimes develop ulcers and sores in and around the mouth. They are not usually serious, but they can be painful and infectious and need to be treated to alleviate the symptoms and prevent their recurrence.

Visiting the dentist

Ulcers or sores that don't clear up easily require a special trip to the dentist. Whether a special or routine visit, try to reassure your child that her treatment will help alleviate pain and keep her teeth healthy.

Mouth ulcers, open sores that commonly develop in the mucous membrane lining the mouth or on the side or underside of the tongue, are painful but rarely serious. The most common type is an aphthous ulcer. These mini-craters sometimes occur in crops and tend to be recurrent. It is not known what causes them.

Mouth ulcers can also be caused by minor injury, for example from a sharp tooth, hitting the gum with a toothbrush or accidentally biting the inside of the cheek. The ulcer usually develops two to three days after the injury. Most ulcers heal without treatment within 4 to 10 days, but the larger the ulcer, the longer it takes to heal.

Sluicing the mouth with a teaspoon of salt added to a glass of tepid water can help relieve pain. There are also several anaesthetic gels available over the counter from pharmacies and, if the pain is severe, your child may be given paracetamol linctus. She should avoid acidic, spicy, hot or salty foods until the ulcer has healed. Drinking through a straw may help.

If an ulcer fails to heal, or if your child experiences recurrent ulcers, the dentist may prescribe a paste, which may sometimes contain hydrocortisone, to cover the ulcers.

Oral thrush

Also known as oral candidiasis, oral thrush is an infection of the mouth. It is caused by *Candida albicans*, a yeastlike organism that lives naturally in the mucous membranes of the mouth and the gut. Normally, the organism is kept in check by bacteria that also live in the mouth; however, if the balance of microorganisms becomes unstable, the yeast grows uncontrollably.

The condition is most common in babies in their first year of life, but older children may be affected after a course of antibiotics. The steroids in inhalers used for treating asthma (see pp.76–77) can also upset the flora of the mouth, leading to thrush. (Inhalers may also cause a dry

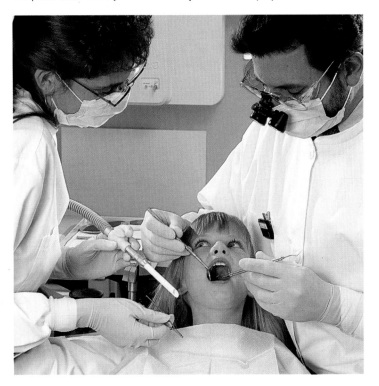

mouth.) Infection with HIV (see p.73), which impairs the immune system, can occasionally be another cause.

Symptoms include a sore mouth, which can make feeding or eating difficult, and a creamy yellow or white coating on the tongue and other areas in the mouth, which cannot be scraped off. You should consult a dentist or doctor, who will examine the child's mouth and may take a sample of the coating for analysis. He will probably prescribe an antifungal preparation that is applied to the mouth. If you are breastfeeding, the doctor may prescribe an antifungal cream or ointment to apply to your nipples too.

To prevent reinfection, you should thoroughly clean all bottles and teats. In children with asthma, the risk of thrush can be reduced by rinsing the mouth or cleaning the teeth after using an inhaler.

Cold sores

Painful blisters, or vesicles, caused by the herpes simplex virus, are known as cold sores. They occur on and around the lips. The virus is common – 50 to 60 percent of adults are infected – and it is often passed from parent to child. Any member of the family with cold sores should use a separate towel and flannel.

The first episode of an infection – or the primary infection – may cause few or no symptoms, but some children experience a flulike illness. In some cases, when a primary infection occurs between birth and three years of age, the child develops mouth ulceration and fever.

Once the child has contracted the virus, she will have it for life. The virus lies dormant in the nerves and may be reactivated at any time, especially if the child is run-down. It can also be triggered by sunlight, wind, colds and other infections that depress the immune system. However, outbreaks will usually become less frequent with time.

When the virus is triggered, the child will usually experience a tingling, itchy sensation a few hours before the cold sore breaks out. Within a few days the skin becomes red and a blister or blisters form. These enlarge and burst, leaving a small raw area. It is at this stage that the virus is most exposed and can be transmitted to other people. The blister crusts over and heals within 10 to 14 days. The blisters can be itchy and unsightly, but they are not usually serious; however, touching the eyes after touching a sore can cause a corneal ulcer, which can lead to blindness.

Using an antiviral cream or ointment available by prescription or from the pharmacy can often prevent a cold sore outbreak from progressing if it is applied at the tingling stage. It is much less effective after the blister has started. If a cold sore does develop, keep your child's hands clean and encourage her not to touch the sore. She should also not kiss anyone, especially other children, until the cold sore has healed. If the sore is painful, a cold drink or ice lolly can often help. Using sunblock on your child's lips can help to prevent cold sores that are triggered by sunlight.

SEE ALSO

Bottlefeeding	33
Teeth and tooth care	38–39
Leukaemia	117
The mouth and teeth	150–151

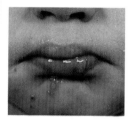

Cold sores in babies
A cold sore makes it difficult and painful for a baby to suckle. Nipples, bottles and teats must be kept clean, and an antiviral cream used.

GUM-RELATED PROBLEMS

In adults, plaque that is not removed by daily brushing hardens to form calculus (scale), or tartar. This, in turn, can cause gingivitis, inflammation of the gums, which become red, swollen and tender and bleed when brushed. Gingivitis is less common in children than in adults because calculus does not normally form in children; however, in rare instances a tendency to form calculus can be inherited and several children in the same family may suffer from some gingivitis. If this is the case, proper brushing can help prevent it. Regular check ups will ensure that the problem does not return.

Bleeding gums may, rarely, be one symptom of leukaemia. In this case, there are likely to be other symptoms such as pallor, lack of energy and the tendency to bruise easily.

The urinary system and the genitals

Because of the proximity of the urinary system and the reproductive organs, or genitals, sometimes an infection can spread from one part of the body to the other.

Drinking water

Thirst is the body's way of regulating water intake. However, if your child becomes excessively thirsty, consult your doctor.

The main organs of the urinary system are the kidneys. They act as filters by cleansing the blood of waste products, which are excreted in urine. Among the kidneys' other roles, they regulate the volume of the blood and help to control blood pressure. Every minute, large arteries from the heart deliver about a quarter of the blood pumped out by it to the kidneys. Each kidney contains more than a million tiny filtering units, knots of capillaries known as glomeruli, which filter water and waste products from the blood. There are holes in the walls of the glomeruli that act like tiny sieves. If the kidneys are infected and the glomeruli become inflamed, the sieving mechanism does not work and larger molecules escape into the urine, including the protein albumin. When albumin is in the urine, it is a common sign of urinary infection or faulty kidney function.

The antidiuretic hormone (ADH), which is produced by the pituitary gland, determines the concentration of urine. When ADH is present in the blood, a lot of water is reabsorbed into the blood. When the hormone is switched off (see p.133), more water is lost in the urine. In diabetes insipidus (see p.137), ADH is lacking, which causes the production of a large volume of urine. This fluid has to be replaced by drinking plenty of water.

Urination

Urine drains from the kidneys through the ureters (essentially a pair of tubes) into the bladder – the hollow, muscular sac where urine is stored. The bladder stretches and contracts, depending on the amount of urine it contains. Where the ureters join the bladder, they contain one-way valves that prevent urine from flowing back toward the kidneys. The kidneys pass an almost continuous trickle of urine down the ureters. This is stored until the bladder is nearly full, at which point receptors in the bladder trigger nerve messages to the brain, telling you that you need to urinate.

Urine is passed out of the body through the urethra, which is normally kept closed

The urinary system

The kidneys lie at the back of the abdomen on either side of the spinal cord. Tubes called ureters run from the kidneys to the bladder. Another tube, the urethra, extends from the bladder to the outside of the body.

Ureter — Kidney

Bladder — Urethra

COMPOSITION OF URINE

A major function of the kidneys is maintaining the correct balance of chemicals in the blood by excreting toxic substances. Urine consists of 95–96 percent water; the rest is composed of these toxic substances. Urea accounts for 2 percent of urine; sodium chloride (salt), for 1 percent; and other wastes, such as uric acid and creatinine, make up the remainder.

by a sphincter muscle. A boy's urethra is about five times as long as a girl's. During urination the sphincter relaxes and the muscles of the bladder wall contract, causing urine to be expelled. In babies, urine is emptied from the bladder by an automatic reflex; however, with toilet training, this reflex is gradually suppressed as urination comes under the conscious control of the brain. If the urge to urinate occurs when it is not convenient to empty the bladder, the brain sends an order to the sphincter muscle to remain closed.

Newborn babies' bladders are small and, for the first two months, the kidneys are unable to concentrate urine, causing them to expel it 5 to 40 times a day. By two months of age, a baby expels 400 ml (14 fl oz) of urine a day. This gradually increases until, by puberty, the child expels about 1.5 litres (2¾ pints) a day – the same amount as an adult.

The genitals

In girls, the reproductive organs include the uterus, which sits underneath the bladder; the ovaries, where eggs are produced; the Fallopian tubes, which link the ovaries and the uterus; and the vagina, which is the passageway between the uterus and the vulva – the opening to the exterior. Girls normally have a discharge

from the vagina, and it should not be confused with an infection. However, because the urethra is shorter in a girl, an infection from the genital area can more easily spread to the bladder. This includes bacteria that are naturally found in the digestive system, so you should always encourage your daughter to wipe from front to back after going to the toilet.

In boys, the urethra connects the bladder to the meatus, a hole at the tip of the penis – part of the male's reproductive system. The penis hangs in front of the scrotum, the bag of skin that contains the testes, which is where sperm are formed. The tip of the penis, the glans, is protected by a loose fold of skin called the foreskin, or prepuce, an area which should be regularly cleaned to avoid infection.

SEE ALSO

Enuresis	156–157
Problems of the testes	160–161
Urinary tract infections	162
Vaginal problems	163

Male and female systems
Girls have a smaller bladder than boys, and the opening of their urethra lies in front of the vagina (top). In boys (bottom), the urethra passes through the prostate and opens at the tip of the penis.

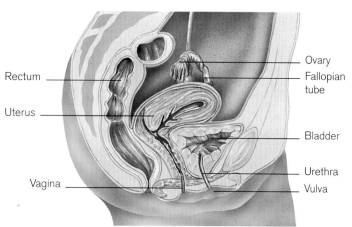

Rectum — Ovary — Fallopian tube — Uterus — Bladder — Vagina — Urethra — Vulva

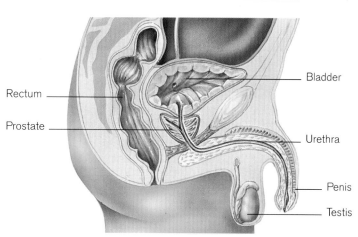

Rectum — Prostate — Bladder — Urethra — Penis — Testis

Enuresis

The medical word used to describe bed-wetting is enuresis, although, strictly speaking, the correct term is nocturnal enuresis. The condition is extremely common, especially among boys.

At the age of 5, about 10 percent of children will wet their bed as they sleep, and even when these children reach the age of 10, approximately half of them will still wet their bed. The condition appears to be more common in some families.

The causes

Enuresis has many causes. It may be a result of delayed maturation of the part of the nervous system that controls the bladder. By the age of 15 months, a toddler will almost certainly be aware of passing urine, although conscious urination is not yet under his control. By 18 months, most toddlers can usually hold urine in the bladder for about two hours. On average, by the age of two a child develops the ability to urinate voluntarily during the day, although complete night-time control is not typical before he is four years old.

Sometimes enuresis develops because of psychological stress or anxiety, a urinary tract infection or diabetes. More rarely, the condition can be caused by a congenital defect of the urinary tract or another condition such as spina bifida (see p.170).

Remember, it is not your child's fault if he wets the bed, nor should you blame yourself. Getting angry or punishing your child may only make the problem worse by inducing anxiety, which is itself associated with enuresis.

Getting a diagnosis

Take a child over five years old who is bed-wetting to a doctor, but if you are concerned about bed-wetting in a younger child, discuss your worries with your doctor, health visitor, school nurse or a continence adviser. It is important to seek help quickly if your child has suddenly started wetting the bed after being dry at night for some time – this could be a sign of a problem such as a urinary tract infection or diabetes (see pp.137–139).

The doctor will ask you and your child (if he is old enough) questions about when the wetting started, how often it occurs and whether there are anxieties at school or home, which may provide clues to the cause. In some cases, the doctor may perform a physical examination, take a urine sample for testing (urinalysis) and carry out other investigations such as an ultrasound scan or an X-ray of the urinary system. Older children who have daytime wetting may be given a bladder function test, or cystometry.

Medical treatments

The doctor will prescribe antibiotics if the problem is caused by a urinary infection, or do further tests if it is associated with other symptoms that could suggest diabetes. Where no physical cause is

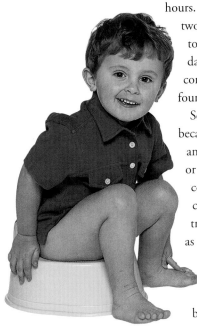

Daytime toilet training
Encouraging a toddler to use a potty at frequent intervals will help him to develop his ability to control urination.

apparent, the doctor may suggest you keep a simple chart with your child of which nights are dry and which are wet. This often improves matters; if not, an enuresis alarm (see below) may be suggested – this is effective for most children. If these measures fail, a doctor may prescribe a drug. Sometimes the child may be referred to a special enuresis clinic, which can provide help, even when no physical cause is found.

Helping your child

Encouragement and support, together with practical measures, can do much to help your child to become dry. Always praise him if he has a dry night, but do not scold him if he has an accident. Sometimes letting your child stick stars on the chart when he has a dry night is helpful, but this may discourage some children if they do wet the bed.

It is important that your child learns to recognize the feeling of a full bladder, so you should encourage him to drink plenty of fluid during the day. Constipation can contribute to bed-wetting, so make sure your child consumes a diet rich in fruit, vegetables and cereals, and that he gets enough to drink. Avoid giving him fizzy drinks, tea, coffee or chocolate before he goes to bed – they contain caffeine and can increase urine production as he sleeps.

Make sure your child urinates before going to bed, and leave a dim light on so that he can find his way to the bathroom easily if necessary. If he wears a nappy at night, he may be less motivated to stay dry, but make sure the mattress is well protected if he goes without one. Ask him to help you change the bed and his nightclothes if he wets himself – this will help him to overcome the problem.

Children over seven years old often benefit from using an enuresis alarm or buzzer. One type consists of a small noise box, which is pinned to the child's nightclothes, and a sensor that is placed between two pairs of briefs or inside a small pad. In the second type, a sensor mat is placed beneath the bottom sheet and the noise box stands beside the bed. In both, the buzzer rings when urination begins, waking the child, who stops urinating and gets up to use the toilet. In time, he learns to wake when he needs to urinate without the need for the alarm.

SEE ALSO

Constipation	**96**
The urinary system and the genitals	**154–155**
Urinary tract infections	**162**

Avoiding stress

Stress from school or in the home can cause bed-wetting. Try to be patient with your child.

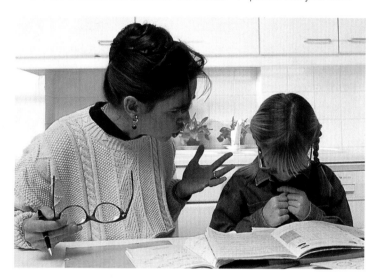

DAYTIME WETTING AND SOILING

If your child starts to wet himself after a period of being dry, there may be several explanations. In a young child, an illness or disruption of his usual routine, such as a holiday or going into hospital, may have provoked the problem, or a urinary infection may occasionally be to blame. In an older child, there may be more deep-seated emotional difficulties. Patience and encouragement will usually solve the problem, but if it continues, you should consult the doctor.

Soiling – accidentally passing faeces – after the age at which bowel control is achieved (usually at about three or four years old) may accompany enuresis. More than half the children who soil also wet the bed. Causes include constipation, slowness to develop bowel control, inadequate toilet training and stress or anxiety. Where there is a physical cause, such as constipation, the soiling usually stops once the problem is treated. If the cause is psychological, simply talking to the child in order to identify what is worrying him may be sufficient; in some cases, however, the child may benefit from being referred to a child psychologist.

Problems of the penis

The urethra runs through the penis and exits at the tip of the penis. A loose fold of skin – the foreskin – covers the glans. Problems can occur if the penis becomes infected or is congenitally malformed.

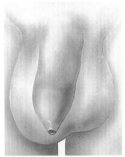

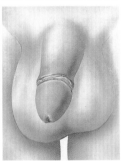

Circumcision

When the foreskin is left intact there is a narrow opening at the tip of the penis (top). On a circumcised penis the glans is exposed (above).

There are certain medical conditions that may require circumcision, the surgical removal of the foreskin, or other surgery. If balanitis, an inflammation of the glans, recurs often or if the child has phimosis or paraphimosis, the doctor may recommend circumcision. In some countries circumcision is performed for religious reasons – for example, if the child is Jewish or Muslim. In the United States, many male babies are routinely circumcised for hygienic reasons.

If you notice any of the following symptoms, your child should see a doctor:
● Difficulty retracting, or pulling back, the foreskin after the age of four years
● Ballooning of the foreskin when the child urinates
● A narrow stream of urine
● A tendency to develop recurrent urinary infections
● A tendency to develop recurrent inflammation and infection
● The urethra opening on the penis is in an abnormal position (hypospadias).

Undergoing surgery

If your newborn baby is circumcised, for medical or other reasons, it may be performed using local anaesthesia. However, in older children it is performed under general anaesthesia. The inner and outer layers of the foreskin are carefully cut off and a small circle of soluble stitches are inserted to hold the raw edges together. These will dissolve over the next one to four weeks. If the foreskin has never retracted, there is likely to be considerable swelling and inflammation.

Surgery to correct hypospadias may take place before the child is two years old, or between the ages of two and four. It may be performed in several stages. The surgeon may construct a tube of skin

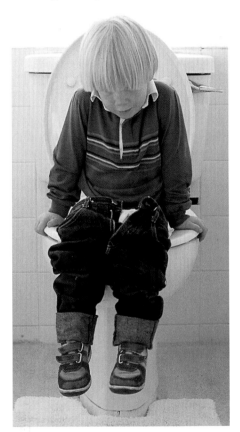

When sitting down is necessary

A boy with hypospadias may find it difficult to urinate from a standing position. He'll have to sit on the toilet until the condition is resolved.

taken from the foreskin or sometimes the bladder lining to extend the urethra so that its opening is in the correct position. If the penis is curved the surgeon will also straighten it. After treatment, the penis will look and perform normally and your son should have no problems passing urine or having sex as an adult.

Regularly bathing your child in salt water will help the wound to heal. There is no need to apply creams or antiseptics unless advised to do so by the doctor. The site may bleed a little during the first week after the operation; however, if it persistently oozes blood for more than half an hour, report it to your doctor.

SEE ALSO

Helping your child in hospital 56–57

The urinary system and the genitals 154–155

COMMON PROBLEMS OF THE PENIS

Condition	Cause/Symptoms	Treatment
Balanitis	A fungal or bacterial infection of the glans – the head of the penis – and the foreskin commonly causes balanitis. Symptoms include swelling of the glans and foreskin in boys who have not been circumcised, pain or itching, redness, moistness and, in some cases, a white discharge. The condition may also be caused by inadequate hygiene or irritation from chemicals in detergents, soaps or bath solutions or from clothing.	Encourage your son to wash his genitals twice a day during and after an attack. If symptoms continue after three days, consult a doctor, who may prescribe an antibiotic or antifungal cream or oral antibiotics. If the condition is caused by an irritation, use a nonallergenic washing product; your son should not use scented soaps or bath preparations. He should wear cotton underwear; thoroughly rinse his clothes in plain water after washing.
Phimosis (tight foreskin)	If the foreskin is too narrow to be retracted, or pulled over, the glans, your son may have phimosis. The foreskin cannot usually be retracted until the age of two, but in some boys this may not happen until they are four years old or older. You should never try to retract the foreskin forcibly, either before or after this age – because you could damage the tissues beneath it, causing bleeding and scarring.	The doctor may recommend circumcision if a tight foreskin causes repeated bouts of balanitis because the area cannot be cleaned (see above) or your son has difficulty passing urine. However, if the foreskin is attached to the glans and the outlet is of a normal diameter, it is possible to separate the tissues surgically without the need for circumcision. This is performed under general anaesthesia.
Paraphimosis	When paraphimosis occurs, it is because the retracted foreskin becomes stuck behind the glans, constricting the penis and causing swelling and pain. It happens if the foreskin of a child with phimosis (see above) is forced to retract.	Take your child to the emergency department. He will be given a sedative or anaesthesia and the doctor will compress the penis so the foreskin can return to its normal position. In some cases, it may be necessary to make an incision to free the foreskin. The condition may recur unless circumcision is performed to correct the original problem – phimosis.
Hypospadias	In 1 in 300 boys, the opening of the urethra is on the underside of the penis, often on the glans – but it can be anywhere on the shaft of the penis. Part of the foreskin may be missing; the shaft of the penis may curve downward, a condition known as chordee. It is not known what causes hypospadias.	The problem is usually detected during a medical examination within the first week of birth. In minor cases no treatment may be needed. However, when the opening is along the underside of the shaft surgery is needed to correct the condition. (Hypospadias can affect a girl – the urethra opens into the vagina – it, too, can be corrected by surgery.)

Problems of the testes

The male reproductive glands – the testes, or testicles – are normally suspended in the scrotum, but sometimes they fail to descend before birth. Other problems are a testis that twists inside the scrotum and swelling.

In about 2 to 3 percent of full-term newborn male babies and 10 percent of premature male babies, one or both of the testes fail to descend into the scrotum. Usually, an undescended testis descends of its own accord within the first year. However, if this does not happen, your child will need medical help.

The testes begin to form within the abdomen of the unborn male baby during the fifth week in the uterus. About two months before birth, the testes normally start to descend into the scrotum, together with the blood vessels and nerves that supply the testes. They finally leave the pelvic cavity by passing through the inguinal canal. This process is stimulated by maternal hormones and by the male hormone testosterone produced by the unborn baby's own testes.

If the hormones fail to stimulate testicular descent, the spermatic cord, which carries the vas deferens and blood vessels to the testis, does not lengthen; this, in turn, prevents full descent. Sometimes the testis is partially descended or it has descended into the wrong place. The testis can also be damaged before, during or after birth. This may happen if the spermatic cord, from which the testis is suspended, twists (see Testicular torsion, opposite) and obstructs the blood circulation to the testis – without a blood supply the testis dies. Rarely, the testis fails to form altogether.

An undescended testis will not develop normally and cannot produce sperm. If both testes remain undescended, the boy is likely to grow up infertile. Undescended testes are also linked to an increased risk of testicular cancer. However, early treatment will help to improve the child's chances of being fertile.

Diagnosis and treatment

The condition is usually picked up during the routine medical examination that every newborn baby undergoes within a few days of birth. In certain cases, diagnostic tests, such as ultrasound, may be carried out.

Injections of the pregnancy hormone hCG (human chorionic gonadotropin) may be given, which causes the testis to descend in about 30 percent of boys. However, in one-third of these cases, the

How the testes descend

The testes develop near the kidneys in a foetus. Normally, shortly before birth, they move down the inguinal canal into the scrotum.

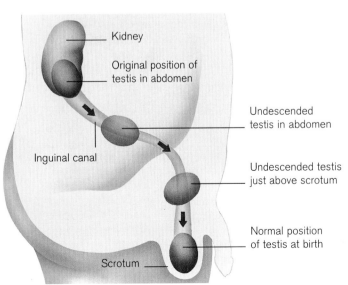

Kidney

Original position of testis in abdomen

Undescended testis in abdomen

Inguinal canal

Undescended testis just above scrotum

Normal position of testis at birth

Scrotum

EXPLAINING TO YOUR CHILD

If your child has undescended testes, you need to provide him with a simple explanation of his condition and any treatment that he may need. Tell him that his testis (or testes) did not come down into his scrotum, as it (or they) should have, when he was inside your tummy. Explain that this means he may have trouble when he grows up and that he needs to have an operation to bring the testis into the proper position so that he will be able to have children of his own one day.

Tell him that before the operation the doctor will give him special medicine to make him go to sleep so that he will not feel anything. Reassure him that, although it may hurt a bit after the operation, he will be able to have tablets to take away most of the pain.

effects of the hormone treatment are not permanent and surgery is the only option.

The most common treatment is orchidopexy, an operation that brings the testis down into the scrotal sac. There is some evidence that younger children tolerate the discomfort of surgery better than older children, and the operation is generally performed when the child is two or three years old.

The child is given general anaesthesia and an incision is made in the groin. A laparoscope, an instrument with a lens at the end of a tube, may be used to identify the site of the undescended testis. When the surgeon has located the testis, he gently frees it and moves it down into the scrotum. The base of the testis is usually attached to the scrotum with stitches to prevent it from retracting. The child will be given painkilling drugs to alleviate pain and swelling.

If the undescended testis is found to be poorly developed, and the other testis is

normal, the surgeon will remove the immature testis. This procedure is known as an orchidectomy.

Hydrocele

A hydrocele is a soft, painless swelling in the scrotum caused by fluid around the testes. The condition is common in newborn babies and the testes appear unusually large. It usually disappears by the time the child is about six months old without the need for treatment.

Sometimes, however, a hydrocele is associated with an inguinal hernia (see pp.94–95), which may need surgery to correct it. In older boys a hydrocele may be caused by inflammation, infection or injury, and if it occurs, you should take the child to see the doctor.

The doctor will examine your child and may order investigative tests, such as an ultrasound scan, to make sure the testes are not damaged. If the hydrocele does not disappear and the swelling is causing discomfort, the fluid can be drawn off under local anaesthesia.

TESTICULAR TORSION

In this condition, the testis rotates and twists the spermatic cord and blood vessels running alongside the cord, eventually cutting off the blood supply. This causes irreversible damage to the affected testis if left untreated. The child may be slightly feverish, the testis will be swollen and tender, and that side of the scrotum will appear red and inflamed.

Some 20 percent of twisted testes occur in newborn babies and show up as a discoloured scrotum. The next peak incidence is at puberty, when testicular torsion frequently causes lower abdominal, rather than testicular, pain – it is important, therefore, to examine this area in boys with unexplained abdominal pain.

The child will need urgent referral to a paediatric surgeon, who will explore the area and untwist and save the testis if possible. Both testes are then anchored in the scrotum with stitches to prevent further torsion. If the doctor does have to remove one testis, the child will be able to function perfectly well with the other one, and if it is thought advisable, a prosthetic testis can be inserted into the scrotum at a later date.

Urinary tract infections

Such infections are particularly common in girls and newborn baby boys. The infection is usually caused by bacteria and can affect any part of the urinary system – the urethra, the bladder or the kidneys themselves.

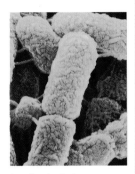

Invading bacteria

The *Escherichia coli*, or *E. coli*, baterium, which normally lives harmlessly in the rectum, is the culprit responsible for about 80 percent of urinary tract infections.

Urinary tract infections (UTIs) usually occur when bacteria that normally live harmlessly in the rectum travel, via the urethra, into the urinary tract, where they breed. Girls are more prone to infections than boys because their urethra is shorter and closer to the rectum.

Symptoms

In an older child, symptoms include pain or burning on passing urine; wanting to urinate frequently but being able to pass only a dribble; bed-wetting or daytime wetting after a period of being dry; and discoloured, cloudy or smelly urine. The child may complain of low abdominal or back pain and she may have a raised temperature. In a young child or baby, symptoms may be less specific such as a raised temperature, irritability, listlessness, possible diarrhoea or vomiting and strong-smelling urine.

Diagnosis and treatment

If you suspect your child has a urinary infection, take her to the doctor at once. If she is old enough to provide a midstream urine sample, take it with you in a sterile container. The urine will be checked to see whether or not there is an infection and, if so, which bacteria are causing it. If there is an infection, the doctor will prescribe a course of antibiotics, after which the child's urine will be tested again to make sure that there are no remaining bacteria.

The doctor may refer your child to a specialist to be tested for scarring of the kidneys or congenital abnormalities of the urinary tract.

Avoiding urinary tract infection

To prevent recurrences, your child should:
- Drink plenty of fluids
- Pass water at regular intervals
- Empty the bladder completely – after passing urine, tell her to count to 20 and to try again to get out the last drops
- Wipe the bottom from front to back
- Avoid constipation
- Bath or shower every day, using nonallergenic soap
- Wear cotton underwear.

KIDNEY INFECTIONS AND DIALYSIS

Repeated kidney infections or serious kidney disease may damage the kidneys, causing renal failure. The kidneys are unable to make urine, so wastes accumulate in the bloodstream. Left untreated, this is fatal. Symptoms of serious kidney disease include poor growth; excessive thirst, especially at night; passing abnormal quantities of urine (too much or too little); abnormalities of the urine such as blood or frothiness; and a puffy, swollen face or feet because fluid accumulates in the tissues.

Many children whose kidneys have failed can be helped by dialysis, in which the blood is cleansed by a machine. There are two methods. In hemodialysis, blood is passed through an artificial kidney machine. In peritoneal dialysis, the waste products are removed using the body's natural filtering membrane, the peritoneum, which lines the abdomen. The dialysis is usually performed overnight so the child can be up and about during the day. Complete kidney failure is rare, but if the kidneys have failed permanently, dialysis will have to be performed in the hospital until the child can have a kidney transplant.

Vaginal problems

An unusual discharge and itching around the vagina are uncomfortable conditions that may affect girls from the time they are babies. It is important to help your daughter deal with such sensitive problems without embarrassment.

The most common cause of vaginal discharge is thrush, which is usually accompanied by soreness, redness and itching. Babies can contract the infection, which is caused by the yeastlike organism *Candida albicans*. The organism lives naturally in the vagina, bowel and mouth, where it is kept in control by other bacteria. When this natural harmony is disrupted – for example, by a run-down immune system or when taking a course of antibiotics – the candida organism flourishes and the symptoms develop. Treatment consists of an antifungal preparation in the form of an ointment or cream or taken orally.

A persistent vaginal discharge may sometimes be a result of the girl inserting an object into her vagina that is forgotten or that she is too embarrassed to tell you about. In this event, the object may have to be removed under anaesthesia.

It is possible that a vaginal discharge may be a symptom of sexual abuse. If you suspect this, you should report your suspicions to your health visitor or doctor so that you and your child can get proper help and support.

Vaginal itching

Vulval and vaginal itching may be caused by thrush, but it can also be caused by threadworms, a parasitic infestation of the rectum; by a bacterial infection; by an allergic reaction to soaps or bubble baths; by poor hygiene; or for no other reason than that the girl has sensitive skin. When an infection is present, there will be other symptoms, such as inflammation, soreness and a discharge; there may also be pain on urination. An infection should be treated with the appropriate drug.

When there is no obvious cause, the itching may clear up of its own accord, but if the child scratches, a vicious circle of scratching and itching may be set up. To alleviate discomfort, she should bathe the area twice a day with plain cool water, and apply a soothing cream such as zinc and castor oil. She should wear cotton underwear and change it daily; do not use biological washing powders and always rinse her underwear in plain water.

If the itching is persistent and self-help measures do not cure it, a doctor may prescribe a hormonal cream to thicken the skin of the vaginal area.

MENSTRUATION

During childhood, a girl's ovaries grow larger and secrete small amounts of oestrogen. As puberty approaches, the body begins to release other hormones, which set the ovaries into action. The first menstrual period, known as the menarche, happens on average at age 13. However, the age of menarche has been dropping in recent years and it is not unusual for girls to begin having periods when they are as young as 10 or 11 years old.

You should prepare your daughter for the onset of menstruation, explaining why it happens and how she can deal with it using sanitary pads or small tampons that are easier to insert than the regular variety. At the same time you should explain the physical – and emotional – consequences of intercourse, along with the risks of pregnancy and infections and how to avoid them.

The brain and nervous system

The brain is the control centre of the body – with its network of nerves, it senses conditions inside the body and around it, then determines an appropriate reaction.

Nervous system

The network of nerves forms a two-way system. It collects and sends data via the spinal cord to the brain, which then processes the details and returns a response.

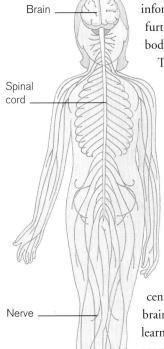

Brain

Spinal cord

Nerve

The nervous system has two main sections: the peripheral nervous system and the central nervous system. The peripheral nervous system contains all the nerves connecting the brain and spinal cord to the rest of the body. It gathers information from different parts of the body and carries it to the central nervous system – the brain and spinal cord – which then interprets this information and responds with further signals instructing the body how to react.

The peripheral nervous system controls basic unconscious activities, such as breathing, digestion and blood pressure, and it collects information from the outside world using sensory organs such as the eyes and the skin. It also controls conscious activities such as walking.

The brain

The major organ of the central nervous system is the brain. Scientists still have a lot to learn about how this complicated organ works. Most of its growth and development occurs in the first five years of life. By the time a newborn reaches 12 months of age, her brain will have doubled in weight. This is why the bones in the skull do not fuse together until the age of six (see pp.10–11).

The brain is most active under the age of three, which is when it has the greatest capacity for learning. This is also when the brain establishes a pattern for the basic ways of thinking, responding and solving problems – so this is the age at which you and those around your baby, along with her environment, will have the most influence on how she develops.

A brain injury at any age can cause permanent damage, but a child can recover better than an adult because her brain is more adaptable – the function of the damaged part of the brain is more likely to be taken over by another part.

Working in harmony

The brain has three regions: the brain stem, cerebellum and cerebrum. These are divided into distinct areas, each of which has its own functions but also works in harmony with the other regions. The brain stem acts as a pathway for all the nerve messages going in and out of the brain. It controls automatic activities vital for life such as the heart rate, blood pressure, swallowing and consciousness.

The cerebellum processes information from the part of the brain that directs movement, or motor activities, sending out messages to maintain balance and posture and ensure coordinated muscle movements at a subconscious level.

HOW PAIN IS FELT

A complex sequence occurs when a child reacts to pain such as when she burns a finger.

1. Sensory receptors receive messages from the heat source and transmit them via a sensory nerve to the spinal cord.

2. From there, a signal travels via a motor nerve concerned with movement back to a muscle, which contracts to move the finger away from the heat. This is a reflex arch.

3. Other signals are sent to the cerebral cortex, where the child perceives the sensation of pain. The signals may be reinforced by other sources such as what her eyes see.

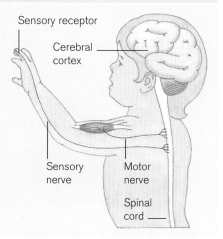

Sensory receptor

Cerebral cortex

Sensory nerve

Motor nerve

Spinal cord

The cerebrum has two hemispheres, and the entire surface is covered by wrinkled grey matter, the cerebral cortex. The cortex is divided into several lobes, and each is linked with specific activities. For example, the temporal lobes are responsible for hearing and smell, and the parietal lobes are concerned with touch and taste. The cerebral cortex processes and analyses information from our senses, enabling us to communicate, think, remember and perform conscious activity.

The cortex develops differently in girls and boys. The left half of the cortex develops earlier in girls, giving them better language-related skills; however, the right half of the cortex is usually better developed in boys, allowing them greater spatial awareness.

Within the cerebrum are the thalamus, hypothalamus and limbic system. The thalamus transfers information between the spinal cord and the cerebral hemispheres. The hypothalamus is concerned with controlling vital functions such as appetite, thirst, wakefulness and sleep, and temperature; it is linked to the endocrine system. The limbic system controls emotional response.

Protecting the nervous system

The tissues of the brain and nervous system are soft and delicate and can be easily damaged. To protect them, both the brain and spinal cord are covered by three fibrous membrane layers, the meninges. A watery cushion of cerebrospinal fluid circulates among the meninges, the spinal cord and cavities in the brain. It nourishes the brain and nervous tissues and protects them from injury. An outer solid bony casing – the skull, or cranium, in the case of the brain, and the vertebral column, or backbone, for the spinal cord – is the final layer of protection.

New sensations

On his first encounter with snow, a baby introduces new data to his nervous system, which is responsible for interpreting the sensation of cold.

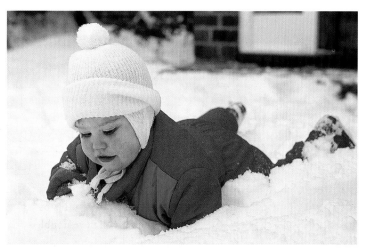

Headaches

Most headaches are usually insignificant, a symptom only of a childhood illness. However, one in five children suffers from recurrent headaches, which are sometimes linked to anxiety, migraine or eyesight difficulties.

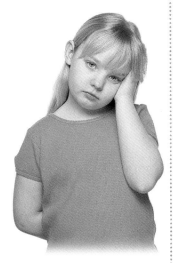

Recurrent headaches

If your child develops headaches after reading a book, she may have a vision problem.

A child with a raised temperature, sinusitis or toothache often has a headache too. Sometimes, a headache heralds the onset of an illness such as measles or influenza. If a headache is accompanied by fever, drowsiness, stiff neck, vomiting, an intolerance of light or confusion, it could be caused by a more serious problem such as meningitis or encephalitis – seek medical help straight away. The child should see a doctor if he has a headache after a recent fall or blow to the head – this is a sign of concussion.

If your child has a headache, check for other symptoms such as an earache, cold or respiratory infection. As long as his temperature is normal, encourage him to get some fresh air. If it has been a while since the child has eaten, give him something light to eat and drink. Give a child paracetamol for a headache that lasts longer than an hour, and let him rest in a darkened room for a short time.

Recurrent headaches

In a child who is otherwise well, stress may cause recurrent headaches (see pp.186–187); give him paracetamol to alleviate the pain and try to discover what is worrying him. If the problems and the headaches persist, your child may be referred to a counsellor or psychotherapist.

If your child experiences recurrent headaches after using a computer, watching television or reading, he may have an eyesight problem (see pp.84–85); take him to a doctor or optometrist.

Some children – especially those who have relatives who suffer from migraine – have recurrent stomachaches and headaches, or abdominal migraine. They are prone to migraines as adults. Older children may experience classic migraine symptoms, with nausea, vomiting and visual disturbances. Your child's doctor can identify potential trigger factors, such as stress, citrus fruit, chocolate, cheese or tiredness, and may prescribe a drug to avert attacks.

Rarely, recurrent headaches indicate something more serious. If they occur in the morning on waking, on both school days and holidays, consult your doctor.

ENCEPHALITIS

Encephalitis is an inflammation of the brain. Often the cause of the disorder is not found, but among the known causes are the herpes simplex virus (see pp.108–109), measles (see p.68), chickenpox (see p.63), whooping cough (pertussis; see p.70), rubella (German measles; see p.71), HIV (see p.73) and many other viruses. Symptoms include headache, fever, confusion, mood changes, disturbed behaviour and convulsions (opposite).

If the meninges, the membranes around the brain, are affected as well, the neck is stiff and the eyes are abnormally sensitive to light. Take your child to a doctor immediately if he has these symptoms. A lumbar puncture, in which spinal fluid is drawn off through a hollow needle, may be done to exclude bacterial meningitis (see pp.66–67).

If the cause of encephalitis is the herpes simplex virus, the drug acyclovir may be given; however, other viruses do not respond to drug treatment. Although most children will recover completely, a small proportion are left with permanent brain damage and, rarely, a child may die.

Febrile convulsions

A febrile convulsion is a seizure induced by a high temperature of 39°C (102.2°F) or above. The condition usually affects 1 in 30 children between the ages of six months and three years.

A young child's nervous system is immature, so it cannot adapt to a sudden change in body temperature. The child loses consciouness, his limbs become stiff or floppy and he may briefly stop breathing and lose control of his bowels or bladder. This may be followed by the child's limbs jerking, and he may froth at the mouth and his eyes may roll back.

When the child regains consciousness, he will probably appear confused or irritable and will usually sleep for several hours. About one-third of children who have one febrile convulsion will have another one. Although alarming, they are not harmful, and most children grow out of them between the ages of three and five. Rarely, some children who have convulsions will develop epilepsy.

Treatment

If your child has a temperature of 39°C (102.2°F) or more, give him paracetamol or ibuprofen, take off his top layers of clothes and sponge him with tepid (not cold) water. If your child has a seizure, place him in the recovery position (see p.213 and p.215). Stay with your child and reassure him once it has passed.

If it is your child's first convulsion, call the doctor or take him to the accident and emergency department. A child is usually admitted to hospital to identify the potential cause and rule out serious causes. The doctor will give you advice on how to deal with future convulsions and may prescribe an anticonvulsant drug to shorten convulsions. Seek medical help immediately if a seizure lasts for more than 5 minutes (or 15 minutes after the drug has been administered) or if one seizure quickly follows another.

FAINTING

A lack of blood supply to the brain can cause fainting – a loss of consciousness. It may be induced by standing for a long time, being in a hot, enclosed space or by anxiety. The child's skin colour will become pale and he may sweat. He may also complain of dizziness and nausea.

If your child feels faint, lie him down with his legs raised on several cushions to increase blood supply to the brain. Open windows to let in fresh air, loosen his clothing and calmly talk to him. A sugary drink or snack such as a biscuit may help if low blood sugar is a problem. However, do not give your child anything to eat or drink if he is not fully conscious. If your child does lose consciousness, lie him in the recovery position (see p.213 and p.215). If your child has not begun to recover within five minutes, get medical help. If he frequently faints, make an appointment to see the doctor.

Reducing a fever
Loosen or remove your child's clothes before you sponge her down, using a flannel soaked in tepid (not cold) water.

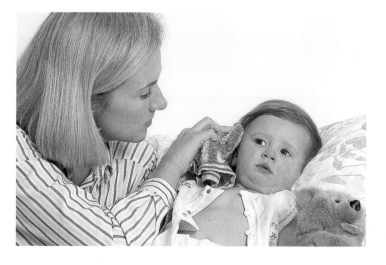

Epilepsy

Of every 200 children, one will have epilepsy, or a tendency to experience recurrent seizures of the brain. They are caused by a temporary episode of uncontrolled brain activity, which is known as a brainstorm.

A seizure can affect the whole of the brain or only a part of it. The most common types of seizure are tonic-clonic (or grand mal) seizures and absence (or petit mal) seizures. About three-quarters of children with epilepsy have tonic-clonic seizures. During a seizure the muscles contract, forcing air out of the lungs, and the body stiffens and jerks uncontrollably.

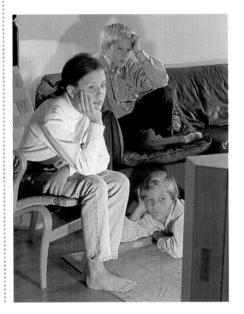

The child may cry out as she falls down unconscious. She will be pale and her breathing may be irregular; she may emit strange sounds, dribble, bite her tongue or be incontinent. Afterward, the child will not remember what happened. She often feels drowsy, confused and has a headache and may sleep for several hours.

An absence seizure can be difficult to diagnose – there is a short absence of awareness that may be misinterpreted as daydreaming. The child stops what she is doing and stares, blinks and looks vacant for a few moments.

Diagnosis and treatment

If it is suspected that your child has epilepsy, she will be referred to a paediatrician, who may order a number of tests such as a computerized tomography (CT) scan or a magnetic resonance imaging (MRI) scan to study the brain.

Seizures are usually controlled by medication, and most children are able to live healthy, active lives. Once the child has been free of seizures for at least two years, the doctor may try to phase out the drugs. If the child's seizures cannot be controlled by drugs, surgery may be an option. Some cases will respond to a vagal nerve implant, in which a device is implanted in the chest to block the nerve impulses that cause seizures. Although many children grow out of epilepsy, some do not and have to continue taking medication for life.

Flashing lights

In a few cases flickering lights from a television screen can trigger a fit. If this is the case for your child, she should watch television in a well-lit room and not get too close. To turn it off, she should use a remote control or approach the television from the side.

TRIGGERS

Some people can identify certain factors that trigger a seizure:
- Stress and anxiety
- In 5 percent, patterns of light from televisions or computer screens, or flashing camera or discotheque lights
- Late nights and lack of sleep
- Illness with a high temperature (see febrile convulsions, p.167).

Cerebral palsy

About 1 in 400 children has cerebral palsy, a disorder
that affects movement and posture. Some children will
have mental difficulties and are slower than average
to learn, but most are of normal intelligence.

SEE ALSO
Caring for a child with
special needs   198–199
Speech and language
problems   200–201

Some children with cerebral palsy are
so mildly affected that it is scarcely
noticeable; others with the disorder have
problems walking, feeding, talking, sitting
up and using their hands. Sometimes
other parts of the brain are affected and
the child has problems with seeing,
hearing, perception and learning. One-
quarter to one-third of children with
cerebral palsy are also affected by epilepsy.

There are three main types of cerebral
palsy. In spastic cerebral palsy – the most
common type – which acts on the cortex,
the muscles are stiff and weak. Athetoid
cerebral palsy affects the basal ganglia in
the brain. The child may find it difficult
to control her posture and may make
involuntary movements with her legs
or arms. Ataxic cerebral palsy influences
the cerebellum. It causes difficulties with
balance, shaky hand movements and
irregular speech. Children may have
a mixture of the different types.

Cerebral palsy often becomes apparent
when the baby is 6 to 12 months old. It
is usually caused by failure of part of the
brain to develop during late pregnancy or
in early childhood. This may be because
of bleeding or blockage of the blood
vessels in the brain, through deprivation
of oxygen during birth or as a result of
prematurity. Low birth weight babies
are most likely to be affected. Certain
infections during pregnancy, such as
rubella (see p.71), or during early
childhood, such as meningitis (see

pp.66–67) or encephalitis (see p.166), may
also lead to cerebral palsy. In rare cases, it
is the result of an inherited disorder.

Treatment

When started from an early age, treatment
can help alleviate the effects of cerebral
palsy. Physiotherapy is the mainstay of
treatment. It can help improve muscle
stiffness and encourage better patterns of
movement. Occupational therapy can help
the child acquire physical and learning
skills; the therapist can also give advice on
equipment and aids to help the child in
daily life. Speech and language therapists
can help the child with feeding, drinking
or swallowing problems and encourage
learning activities that will help her to
acquire language if there are difficulties.

Playing with friends

If your child is only
mildly affected, she will
attend a mainstream
school and lead a full,
independent life. If she
is severely affected, her
educational needs may
have to be catered for
at a special school.

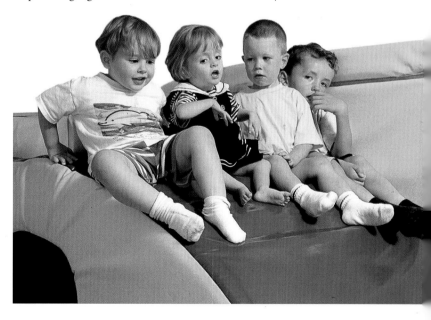

Spina bifida

When one or more vertebrae in the spine fail to form properly, leaving a gap or split, the nervous tissue in the spinal cord is vulnerable to damage or infection – this leads to a disorder known as spina bifida.

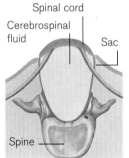

Vertebra

Spinal cord

Nerve

Spinal cord

Cerebrospinal fluid

Sac

Spine

Defective spinal cord

A healthy spinal cord is well protected (top). In one type of spina bifida (bottom), there is a swelling over the spine.

There are several forms of spina bifida and the severity depends on how much nerve tissue is exposed. The mildest type is spina bifida occulta (hidden spina bifida), which may affect as many as 1 in 10 children. It rarely causes any problems or disabilities; in fact, the only visible sign may be a dimple or small tuft of hair on the back. Occasionally, the spinal cord becomes caught against the verterbrae. As the child grows this may affect the nerves that control the child's bladder.

In spina bifida cystica, a sac or cyst covered by a thin layer of skin is visible. In one form, the sac (a meningocele) contains meninges (the membranes that cover the brain) and cerebrospinal fluid. The nerves are often able to function and the child may have little disability.

Myelomeningocele is the most serious type of spina bifida. A sac is visible that contains nerves and part of the spinal cord as well as meninges and cerebrospinal fluid. The spinal cord is damaged or not properly developed, with the result that the child is paralysed and will have little or no sensation below the damaged region. The degree of paralysis depends on where the spina bifida is and the amount of nerve damage. Many children have paralysed legs and difficulties with bowel and bladder control. They may also have cerebral palsy, epilepsy, eyesight problems and learning difficulties.

The cause of spina bifida is still not known, but both environmental and genetic factors are thought to play a part. Taking supplements of folic acid from at least a month before conception to the 12th week of pregnancy can substantially reduce the risk of a baby being born with spina bifida.

If you have given birth to a baby with spina bifida, you are at an increased risk of giving birth to another baby with the condition. Likewise, if you have spina bifida yourself, your risk of giving birth to a child with the disorder is higher. You may benefit from genetic counselling.

Treatment and outlook

If your child is mildly affected, no treatment may be necessary. If he is more severely affected, an operation to close the exposed area in the spinal cord may be carried out to prevent further damage. Physiotherapy and other support can help your child become mobile and live as full and independent a life as possible.

HYDROCEPHALUS

Hydrocephalus affects most babies with spina bifida. The cerebrospinal fluid accumulates in the ventricles inside the brain, causing swelling and compressing the surrounding tissues. The condition may be congenital, and premature babies are at greater risk of developing it. It can also develop from meningitis or a tumour. Left untreated, the child may be developmentally delayed. The outlook is good with treatment, which is to insert a shunt, a device that drains away excess fluid, into the abdomen. The shunt, or a replacement, may remain in place indefinitely. A newer technique, ventriculostomy, avoids using a shunt, but is only suitable in some cases.

Autism

A condition that affects the way a child communicates and relates to other people is known as autism. It can be mild or severe – some children have learning difficulties but others have average or higher intelligence.

SEE ALSO
Identifying a child with
developmental delay   196–197
Caring for a child with
special needs   198–199

Many experts use the term autistic spectrum disorders rather than autism. It is estimated that 2 to 4 children in every 10,000 are affected, and the condition is four times more common among boys than girls. The exact causes of autistic spectrum disorders are still not known, but genetic factors are involved and they may be linked to conditions affecting the development of the baby's brain during pregnancy. The condition is usually evident from birth or before the age of three, although it is not unusual for autistic spectrum disorders not to be recognized until the child is in his teens. Some people with it may even remain undiagnosed for life.

Diagnosis and treatment

There are three impairments to look out for: difficulty with social interaction, social communication and imagination. At the same time the child may exhibit repetitive behaviour and a resistance to change. Children with autism are often slow to learn to talk. They have problems understanding what they hear and a tendency to interpret what people say literally. When a child with autism talks he will tend to talk at others rather than converse with them. The child finds it difficult to express feelings or thoughts and to understand other people's emotions, ideas and thoughts. Some children with autism have some special skills, for example, in music or art.

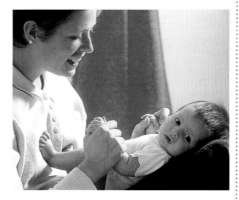

If you suspect your child has autism, make an appointment to see your doctor. He will refer your child to a specialist. Autism is lifelong and there is no single successful treatment. However, with appropriate intervention, specialized education and support, your child may be able to reach his full potential.

Unresponsive baby
One sign of autism in a young baby may be indifference and aloofness in social situations. For example, he may not respond to normal stimulus from his mother.

ASPERGER SYNDROME

One form of autism is Asperger syndrome. A child with the condition exhibits all the typical features of autism, but he has average or above average intelligence. Boys are nine times more likely to have Asperger syndrome than girls. Because he is less obviously disabled than those with "classic" autism, diagnosis is difficult.

He will often speak fluently and may develop an obsessive interest in a hobby or activity. The child may struggle to cope with abstract thinking, which can cause problems with some subjects such as literature, and he may find unexpected changes in his routine particularly upsetting.

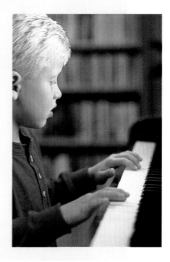

CHAPTER THREE

Behavioural and emotional problems

It is now accepted that a child's mental health needs as much attention as her physical wellbeing. One in five children experiences some kind of emotional upset or behavioural problem. The reasons are numerous and varied, but there is no doubt that the breakdown of the family through divorce and the increased pressure to achieve academic success are important factors.

The earlier a problem is recognized, the sooner a child can be helped. However, it can sometimes be difficult to identify when a child needs help. Parents can often sense that something is wrong but don't know where to go for help. Don't hesitate to seek advice from your doctor, your child's teachers or a parents' support group.

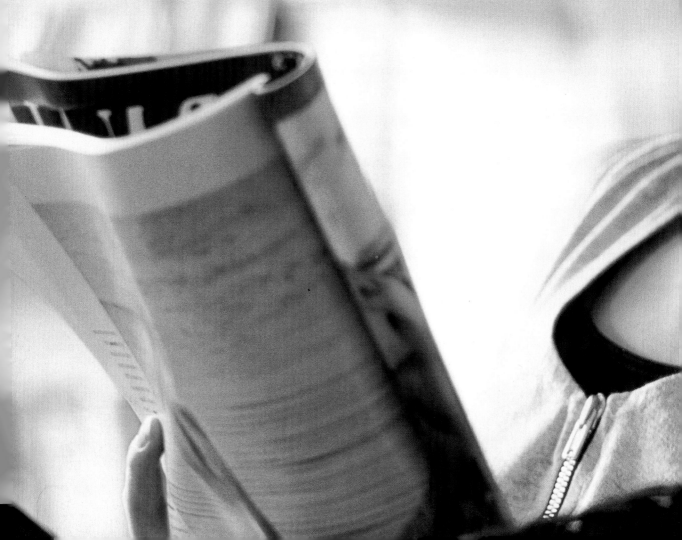

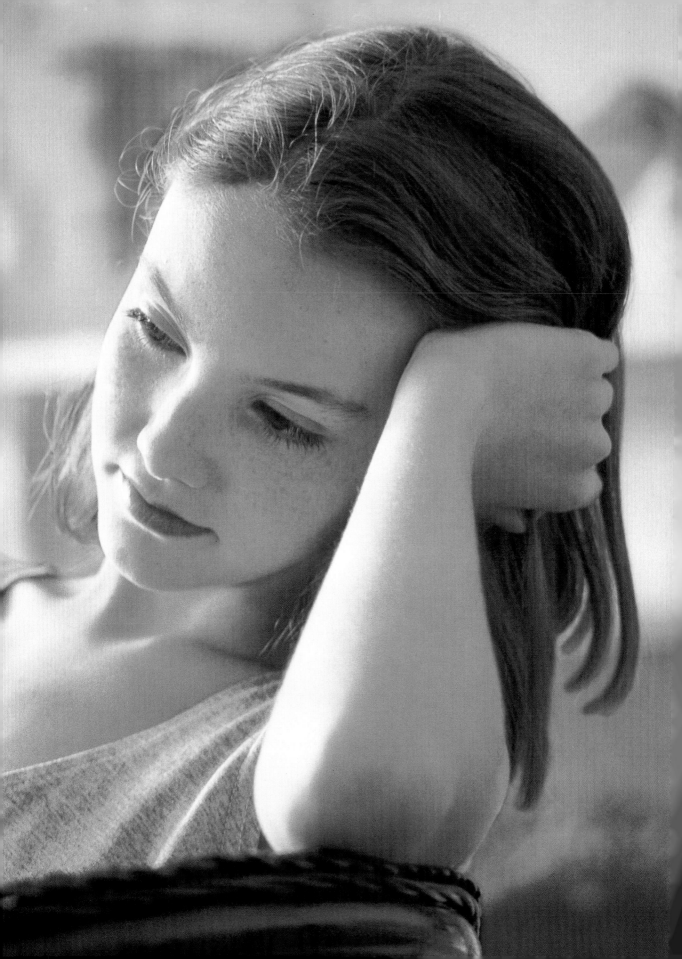

Shyness and insecurity

Although shyness often first appears in young children, even older children who have never shown any signs of being shy before may become so as they reach puberty, particularly with regard to the opposite sex.

Seeking shelter
Instead of letting your older child retreat behind you, give him gentle encouragement to build his confidence.

Parents can become exasperated with a shy child. Everyone would like to have a child who is lively and sociable, and parents can feel let down if their beloved offspring doesn't join in at birthday parties, never initiates conversation and is monosyllabic when people speak to her. Even when parents are shy themselves, they may try to push the child into social situations against her will, particularly if they feel that their own shyness has prevented them from living a full life. At its most extreme, shyness can be seen as a type of shelfishness – the shy person is thought to be so wrapped up in herself that she has no interest in anyone else.

Shyness need not be considered an affliction. It isn't a crime not to enjoy parties, and if your child tends to prefer to play with just a couple of friends who share her interests, there is no need to worry. There are always going to be quiet, passive children, and often they team up happily with friends who are more boisterous and outgoing.

While you cannot change your child's temperament, she is likely to become less shy and wary of social situations when her self-esteem is intact. As a parent you can help her to be more confident by encouraging interests or new hobbies that will give her something to talk about in company. However, if your child's shyness is so crippling that she cannot live a normal life, she may need professional advice.

Insecurity

Giving your child a sense of security is the foundation of good parenting. Knowing that your love is unconditional and that you will always be supportive will help her to face the world and any difficulties she encounters with equanimity. An insecure childhood can often lead to serious mental health problems in later life.

Consistency of care helps a child to feel secure. Children whose carers change on a regular basis – whether it be nannies, child minders or foster parents – often exhibit serious behavioural difficulties. Parents who openly disagree on their child's upbringing and counteract each other are also likely to end up with a confused and insecure child.

Parents should also guard against becoming overprotective. A child must be encouraged to develop independence and self-reliance or she will feel insecure without you in the big outside world.

Comforters

Many babies and small children have a comfort object, which they cling to when they are tired or distressed. This is a familiar possession that gives the child a sense of security. It is usually something

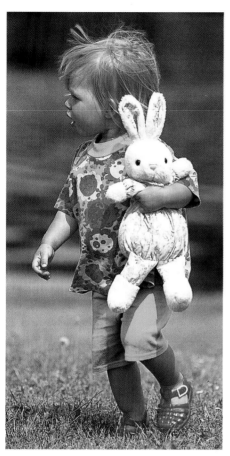

A toddler's best friend

A soft toy, such as a stuffed animal, and a cot blanket are the most common items that children adopt as a comforter.

soft, smooth and suckable, and it will have developed its own comforting, distinctive smell. It may help your child to recall what it was like being a tiny baby, nestling in your arms. While comforters are usually abandoned by the time the child is five or six years old, some children hang on to the object throughout childhood, even if they are careful not to be seen in public with it. If a comfort object is taken away too soon, the child may start sucking her thumb, a habit that can persist into the teenage years. Big children may continue to suck their thumb to help them to fall asleep.

Fears

A healthy reaction to danger is fear. The special fears that small children experience are related to their lack of knowledge of or misunderstandings about the world around them, and these should never be belittled or ignored. Young children do not always have the words to express why they are frightened. The fear may be caused by something in a story you have read together or that she has seen on television. If she constantly asks the same question, then there is something troubling her. One approach is to explain to her that, although you understand why she is scared, she doesn't need to be scared. Or use toys or drawings to play out her fear, which may desensitize her.

Most children enjoy being scared by fairy tale characters such as witches. Such stories can be beneficial, helping small children experience fear in safety. There is some evidence that a child finds stories more frightening on film because the characters move and talk and cannot be controlled by her imagination.

Older children can become fearful of real life events such as a child abduction or major disaster they have seen on television or read about in the newspapers. Gently encourage your child to confront it.

SEE ALSO
Promoting your child's
development: ages 5–12   52–53
Reaching puberty   28–29
Stress and bullying   186–187

Feeling left out

A shy child may become lonely, especially when moving to a new town. Encourage her to join clubs and activities, where she may meet new friends.

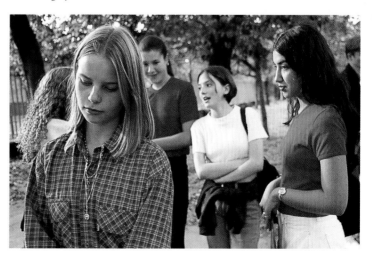

Jealousy and sulking

Most children in a family are likely to experience jealousy, especially when a new baby is born. This may be followed by sibling rivalry, squabbling and sulking – all of which demand a level-headed approach from you.

Almost everyone has experienced jealousy at some stage. Ask yourself how many times you have encountered this feeling, in the workplace or with friends or neighbours. Consider how much more intense it can be in the family and you'll understand and, hopefully, empathize with your child's feelings.

When it comes to your own children, there is a temptation to deny that they could be feeling such negative emotions because it seems to cast you in a poor light as a parent – if they feel this way you must be doing a poor job. This is not the case. If the jealousy is manifesting itself due to the arrival of a new baby, it is perfectly natural that the older child should feel he will never have the same relationship with you again because of the interloper; in truth, this is the case.

It is for you to make him see, through your actions rather than words, that you still love him as much as you did before, but that now there will be more fun because you are more of a family. This is not easy when you are tired from the increased load of parenthood, and it will not happen over night. But most experienced parents will tell you that things will eventually settle down and the jealousy will subside to the point where the first child can't even remember what things were like before the baby was born.

Sibling rivalry

Another entirely normal reaction is sibling rivalry. If you prepare yourself for this particularly annoying and normally recurring emotion in your children, you will not be worn down by it. Remember your own childhood if you had siblings, and acknowledge that the key to handling this is to remain detached and not allow this negative emotion to influence your actions within the home. This is, of course, easier said than done.

When an older child attacks the youngest, who in turn pleads for your intervention, your natural reaction will be to leap in. But it pays to stand back as much as possible. A common aspect of sibling rivalry is that younger children act in a way they know will prompt their older sibling to react aggressively, as a way of securing parental attention. Acting on cue will only teach your younger child to become a victim, and this could lead to his being bullied throughout life. If it really looks like a child will be hurt, insist they both go to separate rooms to cool down, and the key here is to make them both go. Above all, avoid laying blame

Preparing for a new sibling
To help prepare a child for a new sibling, involve her in your pregnancy – let her listen to and feel the baby moving inside you. Explain to her that the new child is someone else for her to love and help look after.

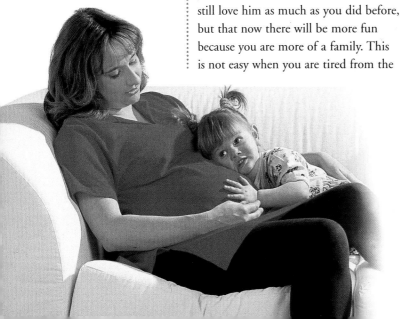

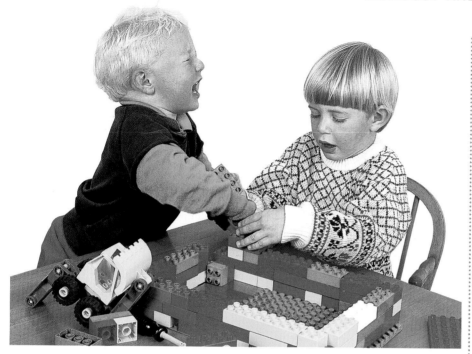

SEE ALSO

Reaching puberty   28–29

Aggression and
tantrums   178–179

Stress and bullying   186–187

A demanding time
Fighting over toys is
common in sibling rivalry,
especially between
younger children. Try
to let them resolve the
conflict themselves.

and don't attempt to sort out every argument in your home. Your refusal to take sides in disputes will eventually signal that their ploys aren't working.

If you notice there is more squabbling going on than normal, spend time with each child individually, and make sure there are no problems from outside the home that could be giving rise to the fight such as bullying at school.

It is important to ensure that older children have space to play without toddler intervention and that younger children are not ridiculed for their games and toys. If one of your children is a talented musician or gifted athlete, don't hesitate to give him moderate praise; but also encourage your other child or children to enjoy different pursuits and praise them for their activities.

Sulking

One irritating means of gaining power and manipulating you is by sulking. It is vital that you consider the underlying feelings that have prompted the sulk rather than becoming angry or feeling threatened yourself. If you have been having coffee with a friend while your child played alongside and this is spoilt by his going into a sulk, you should ask yourself the following questions:
- Could my child feel left out?
- Did I ignore or chastise his efforts to join in our talk?
- Was I talking about him within his hearing?

Be objective and put yourself in your child's shoes. Sulking is an unpleasant tactic, but if your child feels powerless and that his needs are being ignored, he may be acting up as a last resort. If you realize what his grievance is, you need to decide whether it is justified and to modify your actions another time. However, do not change your behaviour as a direct, on the spot, result of sulking, or you will be empowering his negative behaviour. If you recognize some of your own behaviour in your child's sulking, consider some modification, as this is one example you won't want him to follow.

Aggression and tantrums

The transitional stage between babyhood and childhood is often dubbed the "terrible twos" because few children manage to get through this stage without displaying some type of challenging behaviour.

A child throws a tantrum when she is thwarted – either because you have had to refuse her something or because she doesn't have the words to make you understand what she wants or how she is feeling. Perhaps she is tired or hungry, which is often the reason so many children seem to have a tantrum when they are out shopping with a parent.

When a child is having a tantrum, she is often physically strong and may resist all your attempts to pick her up or hold her. Tantrums can be an alarming experience for first-time parents when they find that their happy, easy-going toddler has apparently turned into a monster. Tantrums are easier to deal with when you realize that they are a normal part of development and the result of frustration rather than naughtiness.

It may be helpful to talk to parents who have children of the same age. The best way to deal with a tantrum is to remain as calm as you can. She will only imitate your behaviour if you yell at her. Put some distance between you and your child – take her to another room, if possible, and insist she stays there until she is calmer, being careful to make sure there is nothing there with which she could hurt herself as she continues her rage. Once she has calmed down, give her a cuddle to show that you still love her even though you don't like her behaviour.

When tantrums persist

Most tantrums cease once the child becomes more articulate and can verbalize her needs and feelings, although they may recur during times of stress. Jealousy of a new baby, for example, can cause a four or five year old to resume tantrums; with sensitive handling, the problem should be only a fleeting one.

However, regular tantrums in later childhood are more worrying and can be disruptive to family life. The behaviour is much more likely to persist if the parents have tended to give in to their child

A typical temper tantrum
The child goes red in the face, clenches her fists and screams or sobs loudly. Invariably, she flings herself down and kicks, and she may bang her head on the floor or against a wall.

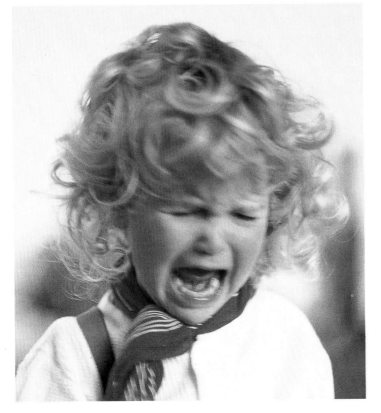

MAKING YOUR CHILD SAFE

If your child is constantly the target of an aggressive child, you need to take action. The first port of call should be her parents, with whom you can work in order to prevent further unpleasant encounters. However, some parents are reluctant to acknowledge bad behaviour in their own child.

If your child is young, then you should be able to avoid any further contact with the aggressive child; but if the incidents are happening away from home, then nursery or school staff must be made aware of what is going on so that they can intervene.

whenever she has thrown a tantrum. When this has previously been such a successful method of getting her own way, there is no reason for her to learn how to negotiate with her parents, as most older children are able to do.

Aggression

In today's society, aggression is very much in evidence, which means that even young children are exposed to it and soon learn to copy this type of behaviour. Parents who have regular displays of bad temper will only encourage their children to behave in the same way. For instance, if they shout and gesticulate at other people when driving, their child will assume that this is the normal way to behave if something annoys them. Aggressive parents will have to learn to control their own behaviour if they don't want their children to imitate it.

Aggressive behaviour is also visible on television and at the cinema, and children do copy what they have seen, as most nursery and kindergarten staff can confirm. Despite the fact that aggression is increasingly tolerated in our society, it

is not an attractive trait and most parents do recognize the need for their child to be taught how to control offensive behaviour and bad temper.

Other children will be frightened of an aggressive child and will try to avoid her, which means she may have difficulty making friends. This can compound the problem – her behaviour is likely to become worse if she is lonely and isolated.

If a child suddenly becomes aggressive, it could mean that her confidence has taken a knock – for example, perhaps she is underachieving at school. This should be discussed with her teachers so that the underlying problem can be identified.

A certain amount of fighting is often tolerated, especially among young boys. Brothers and best friends frequently get involved in fights, but this is often just a way of letting off steam and causes no real harm unless they set out to hurt each other. It's better if they can be encouraged to take up a sport that will use up some of their surplus energy in a more constructive way.

SEE ALSO

Jealousy and sulking	176–177
Hyperactivity	180–181
Stress and bullying	186–187
Substance abuse	192–193

DISCIPLINING YOUR CHILD

Within limits, how you discipline your child is ultimately your decision, but do remember that any strategy should match the age of the child. For example, a toddler should be sent to her room for only five minutes – which is about the length of time that she can remember she did something wrong. The following guidelines may help:

- Give encouragement when your child exhibits good behaviour. Rewarding good behaviour is more effective than punishing bad.
- Don't overuse the word no. If a baby is doing something you don't want her to do, distract her by showing her where she can play. Reserve the use of no for when she puts herself in danger.
- Don't shout at a toddler having a tantrum – it will only make her scream more loudly. Remain as calm as you can.
- Don't give in to a toddler's demands, otherwise she won't learn how to control herself.
- Avoid any form of physical punishment – there is growing evidence that it is counterproductive and sets a bad example.
- Use simple terms to tell an older child why what she did is wrong.

Hyperactivity

There's hardly a parent alive who at one time or another has not thought that his or her child may be hyperactive. However, you can be assured that true hyperactivity, although a serious condition, is comparatively rare.

True hyperactivity, or attention deficit hyperactivity disorder (ADHD), can be difficult to diagnose and treat because its symptoms often resemble the behaviour of normal healthy, exuberant children. Also, there is no medically defined level established to indicate hyperactivity to health professionals and parents.

There are traits that may signal hyperactivity. A short attention span and difficulty in completing a task, even if the activity is one your child enjoys, is a classic sign. Mood swings and impulsive behaviour are another indication. Poor sleep patterns, aggressive behaviour and an inability to cope with being thwarted are other signs. Most children will show some of these symptoms at various times, usually because they are overtired or their routine has been upset. However, if a child, despite having a regular, calm home life, exhibits most of these traits, he may be hyperactive.

Coping with an active child

If you are concerned your child may be hyperactive, it is wise to take stock of his lifestyle before you consult a paediatrician. If he is incredibly restless and fidgets a lot now, he may have been an active baby. Try to remember if there were feeding problems. Did he sleep a lot less than your friends' babies? Did he suffer from colic? Although all these can indicate a hyperactive child, you should also consider his home background.

Children who are cared for by a number of adults, some of whom may have differing ideas about discipline, can become confused about their boundaries and appear hyperactive. Ensure that your child has a calm routine and reinforce positive behaviour while trying to ignore negative traits, so that wild and aggressive habits don't become self-fulfilling.

Bedtime rituals and good sleep patterns go hand in hand. If this is your first child, it may be tempting to carry on with your previous lifestyle and simply take your child with you when you enjoy late nights out, but this will not instil good bedtime habits in your child. The hours before bed need to be calm – a bath and cosy perusal

The hyperactive schoolchild
At school, a teacher may notice signs of a child's hyperactivity, especially if the child is in the habit of disrupting other children during lessons.

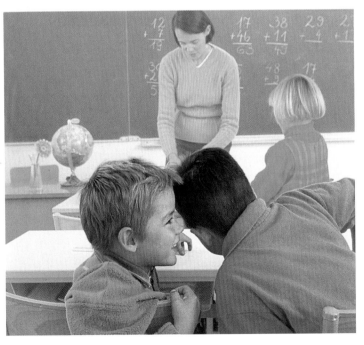

LEARNING DIFFICULTIES

Hyperactivity is often, although not always, accompanied by learning difficulties. These may come about partly through the child's inability to integrate with his peers and teachers and concentrate on given tasks, rather than through low intelligence. Some hyperactive children do suffer from developmental delay to various degrees.

of books together is most likely to help him wind down, especially if he has become overexcited during the day. Persist with this routine for a few months, even if you temporarily miss out socially yourself, in order to ascertain whether your child is exhibiting true hyperactive tendencies or is just in need of a quieter routine.

Many children who appear hyperactive are given no outlet for their energies and are virtually forced to expel them in a negative way, which in turn alienates them from their peers and teachers, and propels the poor behaviour onward. A child who appears overly full of energy can also drain the resources of the rest of the family and upset the balance between siblings and parents, so try to ensure your child is healthily tired by the end of the day.

Swimming sessions or trips to the park may help bring the child's energy levels in line with the other children in the family, although you will undoubtedly need some support if you are not to become exhausted yourself. Try not to rely on television or videos for suppressing his energies because they will only emerge at a later, probably less convenient, time.

Anything you do to pre-empt negative behaviour patterns counts as a positive step away from your child's hyperactive problem. For example, it is worth

considering a parenting course to obtain as many practical strategies as you can for dealing with difficult behaviour. Your health visitor or doctor should be able to advise you about such courses.

When to seek help

Hyperactivity can be caused by an over-active thyroid gland, lead poisoning or a psychiatric disorder, all of which are rare; so you do need to consult your doctor if, despite your efforts, you feel your child's behaviour is still out of control. Your child may be prescribed the drug Ritalin, but the long-term effects are unknown.

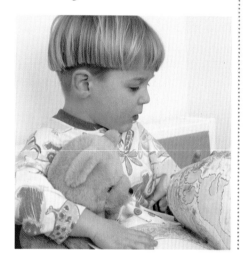

Bedtime ritual
The best way to get your child to sleep is to help him establish a bedtime routine, such as reading a book after he has bathed and changed for bed (see pp.184–185).

SEE ALSO
Thyroid problems   **134–135**
Aggression and tantrums   **178–179**
Stress and bullying   **186–187**

FOOD ADDITIVES

Certain food additives, such as those listed below, may contribute to hyperactive behaviour. If your child is hyperactive, consider excluding these from his diet – they are often found in squashes and sweets.

- Artificial colours: tartrazine (E102); quinolene yellow (E104); yellow (2G E107); sunset yellow (E110); reds (E122–129); patient blue V (E131); indigo carmine (E132); brilliant blue (E133); green S (E142); black PN (E151); brown FK (E154); brown HT (E155); pigment rubine (E180)
- Natural colours: annatto (E160b)
- Preservatives: benzoates (E210–213); sulphites (E220–228); nitrites (E249–252); antioxidants (E310–321)
- Flavour enhancers: glutamate (E621–623)
- Flour improvers: bleaches (E924–926).

Sexual exploration

New parents sometimes become worried about their baby's apparent preoccupation with her sexual organs. This is part of her normal development and is usually no cause for concern.

Starting at about six months of age, a baby may begin to rub her genitals with her hands or against a surface, perhaps rocking backward and forward at the same time – clearly gaining pleasure from the action. This will be the first stage of your baby developing into a normal sexual person.

By the time your child reaches three or four years old, she will begin to display an increasing interest in her own genitals, as well as in those of others. For example, she may ask direct questions about daddy's penis or mummy's breasts. At the same time, she may begin to ask questions about where babies come from. These are normal questions for children of this age, and they should be answered as simply as possible, but with honesty – making up stories will only be confusing.

Also during this stage, your child may become involved in playing doctors and nurses with other children her own age, which usually includes some physical inspection of each other's bodies. Some small children have great fun tickling each other in those sensitive areas. Such inquisitiveness is common to most preschool children and they will outgrow it. This is usually nothing for parents to be concerned about; however, if one child is uncomfortable with this type of intimate playing among a group of friends, then the children should be gently encouraged to play something else. Otherwise, it's best to view the situation as just another learning experience that will soon pass.

Discovering the differences
Young brothers and sisters taking a bath together will often compare anatomical details and comment on the differences between them.

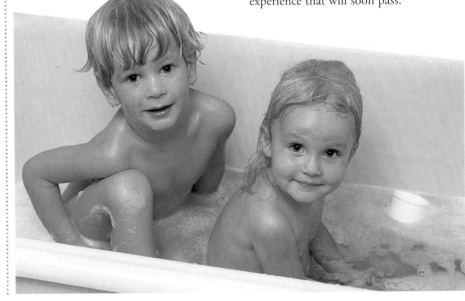

Masturbation

It's inevitable that some parents will feel uneasy about masturbation, and some will be horrified if they discover that their child is masturbating. Some parents may even believe that this is a sign of future deviancy in their child – however, masturbation is common in children of all ages. It does no damage to health; indeed, some people believe that masturbation is a healthy, tension-relieving activity and that children who don't masturbate may indulge in more alarming habits such as pulling their hair.

Even if you have feelings of disgust when it comes to this matter, you should do your best to hide them from your child; overreaction on your part could cause her to develop bad feelings about her own body and can lead to sexual problems in later life. If she does masturbate in public, of course you should distract her, but most children will quickly realize that this is one activity that should take place in the privacy of the home.

When to seek help

There is only need for concern if your child is masturbating constantly and is not doing very much else. First of all, you should have the doctor check her for an infection, which may be causing an irritation that is making her rub her genitals. If that's not the case, then she could possibly be using masturbation as a comfort habit because she's anxious, stressed or bored.

In the early years masturbation is not related to sexual feelings – it only provides a pleasant sensation – but as the child approaches puberty, any time between the ages of 9 and 16, it becomes a normal way of relieving sexual tension for both girls and boys. Boys, in particular, may begin to have sexual fantasies around the age of 11 or 12, and they may masturbate to relieve feelings of frustration.

Sexual development

Your child should be informed – by her parents – about sexuality before the onset of puberty. You may find it difficult to sit down to discuss "the birds and the bees", but research has shown that the fully informed child is more likely to delay the start of sexual activity.

A boy will begin to experience erections in response to some form of sexual stimulation. Once his testes are producing sperm he may be disturbed by involuntary night-time ejaculations, which are often known as wet dreams. His father or other close male relative should reassure him that this is perfectly normal.

A girl who is well developed at an early age may behave in a way that is inappropriate for her age. The danger is that her emotional maturity will not match her physical maturity at this stage. She will need the same protection and support as her less developed friends.

SEE ALSO

Reaching puberty	28–29
Problems of the penis	158–159
Vaginal problems	163
Stress and bullying	186–187

OVERINTEREST IN SEX

A child may become obsessed with sexual matters because she has witnessed adult sexual behaviour or even been the victim of sexual abuse. Sexual abuse of young children is anything ranging from exposure to pornographic material to physical penetration, and it happens in all types of families and in every culture.

Because an abused child is often the victim of someone she trusts, she may think it is something that happens to all children, so the signs of abuse may be detected in her behaviour rather than in what she says, especially if the adult has told her that it is their secret.

Parents and other adults should be alert to the possibility of abuse if a child's role play always has a sexual context, if she draws figures with erect penises and large breasts or peppers her conversation with obscene words. An abused child often behaves in a precocious manner and appears flirtatious. She may kiss other children or adults on the mouth, perhaps even trying to insert her tongue. Behaviour of this kind is a cause for concern for anyone who cares for the child.

Sleeping problems

A baby naps whenever he feels the need, but the parents will suffer from disrupted nights until he learns to adapt to a routine. Sleep problems can recur throughout childhood and should be tackled before they turn into bad habits.

Don't have high expectations that your newborn baby will sleep through the night from the start. Babies under six months of age usually wake at least once a night from hunger, but you should reduce night feeding to a businesslike procedure: keep lights dim or off; avoid talking and prolonged cuddles; only change the nappy if it is soaked through (find a brand that will not need changing or use an extra pad to keep him drier). Gradually, your baby will realize that daytime is the best time to be awake and receiving attention.

If your baby is still waking during the night after six months, you will be feeling the effects and need to develop strategies for getting more sleep. It is important to accept that whatever plans you adopt for

persuading your child to sleep through, it is unlikely to happen immediately; you should prioritize your arrangements to allow you to make up for some of those lost hours. Sleep deprivation can be a serious problem. Make it clear to family and friends that you would welcome any help they care to offer.

Getting your baby to sleep

Establishing a routine may sound like old-fashioned "nanny talk", but it will help him to know what to expect and what is expected of him. Discourage friends from calling in the early evening and avoid going out at night with the baby. Instead, resign yourself to a few months of routine and eventually you will feel energetic enough to go out while a babysitter minds your sleeping child.

Provide a drink or feed, a warm bath, dim lights and a look at his picture books or a few quiet songs. Learn to put your baby down when he is sleepy and relaxed but not already asleep. If he is always put down when asleep, he'll wake and wonder where you are. Ensure that his room is warm – not hot – and that it is dark enough but not pitch black. Keep cot toys to a minimum but put in a mobile or light box for him to fix his eyes on.

For a baby who won't settle down, you can try the "check and leave" routine, which may mean putting up with a lot of screaming. You will need cooperation from your partner and family, and it helps

Crying for a cuddle

It is natural for your baby to feel determined about not staying in his cot when he knows that screaming will elicit a response from you. Establish a routine to teach your child when it is time for him to sleep.

to make a chart to record your baby's sleep progress. To ensure success, you must be firmly committed. Begin when you have a few clear weeks in which you can keep to a routine and not be disturbed by visitors who may find a screaming child upsetting. The success rate for parents using this tactic is high – and before your resolve weakens, remember that long-term disturbed sleep patterns can inhibit your child's growth and development, as well as harm your health.

When your baby screams after he has been put down at bedtime, go to him after exactly one minute. Do not pick him up or establish eye contact. Say some soothing words, stroke him on the head and leave. He will probably scream again, and you will have to repeat your performance after two minutes, then after three minutes, then four. Keep the "check and leave" to every four minutes for three nights. Some babies realize night-time is less rewarding for getting attention and settle quickly after a week. Others resist for longer. During the second and third week you should "check" him every five minutes. This strategy only works if you are completely consistent.

Night waking

Older children can regress to night waking, which can become a habit if you let it. Usually there is a cause that needs identifying. Fears about starting school or other changes to routine can prompt

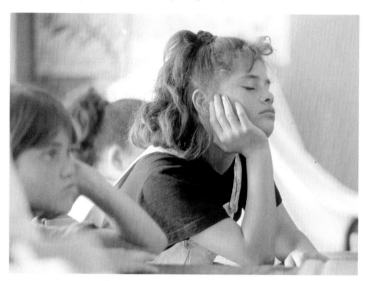

sleeplessness. You can allay your child's concerns through stories or talking.

The amount of sleep that a child needs is variable. Don't trap an older child in the "baby" routine, expecting him to go to bed when he isn't tired. Look for signs of tiredness during the day to determine if he is getting enough sleep, and make time for regular physical exercise. Hours of television or computer games can act as a sedative at the time, only to make the mind overactive at night. If your 10 or 11 year old is sleeping late at weekends, it may be he is catching up on sleep and needs more during weeknights.

SEE ALSO
Bathing your baby and
helping him to sleep   **16–17**
Sudden infant death
syndrome   **18–19**

Daytime napping
If your child's teacher reports that she nods off during lessons, it may be that her sleep is being disrupted by stress (see pp.186–187) or fears (see pp.174–175).

Bedtime nightmares
As a child's mind develops, so does her imagination. If your child has trouble falling asleep because she is scared of the dark, leave a night-light on for her.

Stress and bullying

It is difficult for parents to see their child being placed under undue stress or bullied by peers. To bring an end to these problems, parents need to put aside emotional responses and concentrate on calm, considered actions.

A certain amount of stress can be good; coping with minor stressful situations will make a child better able to handle a more serious stressful situation. However, too much stress can have adverse effects on a child. Research has shown that a child under constant stress has more bouts of colds and digestive upsets and is more likely to be accident prone.

The child's personality, age and previous experiences will all contribute to how she reacts to stress. What might be stressful for one child won't be for another. Common situations that can cause stress are: starting or changing schools, preparing for school exams, not doing well at school, moving and making new friends, parents arguing and family fights, divorce and death of a family member or friend. Pressure from parents for the child to perform better than her ability –

whether in school, sports or playing an instrument – can also cause stress.

Depending on the child, the signs of stress may include:
- Reverting to thumb sucking or bed-wetting (see pp.156–157).
- Irritability and moodiness.
- Becoming aggressive to you or siblings.
- Withdrawal from friends or siblings.
- Worsening performance in school.
- Lack of interest in hobbies or other previously enjoyed activities.
- Sleep disturbances and nightmares.
- Frequent complaints of physical problems such as stomachaches.

As a parent, there are ways that you can help your child. Listen to her and discuss how she feels. Let her know that you recognize that she has to cope with a stressful problem, and share with her your own experiences. Help her to manage the problem by giving her some options. Praise her if she is coping well. Try to avoid compounding stressful situations; for example, don't argue with your spouse in front of her, especially if she is preparing for an important exam.

Bullying

Being the victim of bullying – whether it is name-calling, teasing, exclusion, stealing, hair-pulling, hitting or other physical abuse – is a trying, stressful experience. If your child is six years old or under, she is unlikely to have any qualms about telling you if she is being bullied.

School pressure

By placing too much emphasis on their child getting into the "right" school, parents can make preparing for exams an even more stressful time.

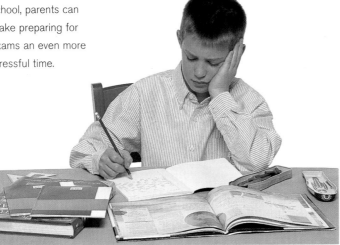

IS YOUR CHILD A BULLY?

For most parents, it is mortifying to have their child accused of bullying or to recognize it for themselves. If this is brought to your attention by your child's school, it is important not to become defensive and offer excuses. Listen to the evidence and take advice.

At home, consider whether your child's needs are met within the family. Those who feel inadequate or have low self-esteem (see pp.174–175), who are bullied by other family members or are victims of some type of abuse, who cannot express their feelings or who come from families where bullying is praised are more likely to be bullies – as are overly spoilt children. If you feel at a loss about how to deal with the problem, consider family therapy.

Before you rush in to protect your child, consider her character. Does she find school difficult? Do siblings often browbeat her? Is she an only child, used to lots of attention? While you should always believe your child, it is not unreasonable to question silently her perception of events. If she has found school difficult, then she may focus on the rough and tumble of the playground. If she is having a hard time with siblings, she may find it easier to complain about children outside the family. If she is your only child, she may be unprepared for the mix of characters that are a part of life outside home. Do not question her too closely, but make an appointment with her teacher when your child will be otherwise occupied.

Children of seven years of age or older are less likely to be open about what is wrong. However, if your child is unhappy and being intimidated, her emotions will surface in the form of stress symptoms (see opposite). She may fake illnesses to stay away from school or avoid taking certain routes to school. Listening to what her friends or other parents say, without resorting to inquisition, and noting the changes in your child are enough to warrant an appointment with her teacher.

Contacting the school

While your child could be the victim of bullying, she may have misunderstood her schoolmates. When visiting the school, make it clear something is wrong, without being accusatory. Your child's teacher should observe your child in class and the playground and report back. If the teacher tells you there are no problems but your child continues to complain, you should persist. Teachers are busy and cannot see everything. You should only remove your child from her school as the last resort if the situation is not resolved. When moved, a child often sees it as a failure in herself and will not necessarily find it easy to settle elsewhere.

You should never show your anger, make threats concerning the bullies or behave in any way that is other than calm. If your child sees how emotional this makes you, she may, unconsciously, use it to seek attention and, unwittingly, place herself in the position of habitual victim.

SEE ALSO

Jealousy and sulking   176–177

Aggression and
tantrums   178–179

Depression   188–189

Poor playmates

Bullies act alone or in a group to single out a child, who is often their own age but may be different – for example, he may be physically weaker than the others or overweight, or he may have an unusual accent.

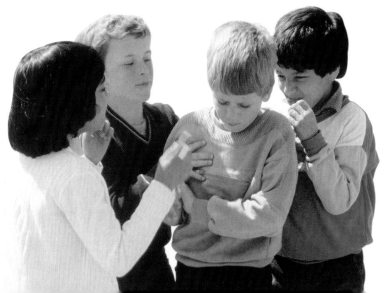

Depression

As much as you would like to, you can't protect your child from some of life's hard knocks – even children may have to cope with depression. With time, your love and support can help him overcome his unhappiness.

Like an adult, a child can have periods of being sad or unhappy, but this does not mean he has clinical depression (see box, opposite). Depression is a complex condition, which varies in its severity. It may be a response to an external factor, such as the death of a family member, which is natural and will subside given time. Or it can be caused by persistent teasing or bullying from siblings or schoolmates, which can be difficult for a child to handle.

An overly anxious child may constantly worry about doing the wrong thing, especially at school. He may become flustered and an underachiever, and he may be upset when a new challenge arises. This type of child often complains about stomachaches and headaches and is easily reduced to tears.

Hereditary factors play a part and if you are a natural pessimist and fearful of what life has in store for you, your child may inherit some of these tendencies, although not necessarily.

How depression manifests itself will vary. An unhappy child may be quiet and withdrawn; however, it is also possible that the child who is badly behaved and disruptive at school may be suffering from depression. Children who are bullies are often those who feel bad about themselves and suffer from low self-esteem. Children with learning difficulties (see pp.206–207) are also more likely to be depressed, as are those with chronic health problems such as diabetes (see pp.137–139) or asthma (see pp.76–77).

If your child seems anxious or miserable for no apparent reason, you do need to be

SEASONAL AFFECTIVE DISORDER

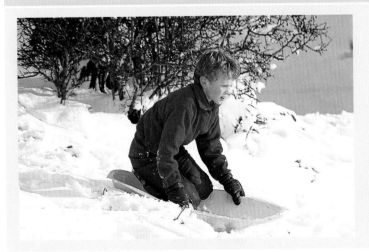

Seasonal affective disorder (SAD), which occurs during the winter months due to the lack of bright sunlight, has been identified in children as young as seven years old. If your child is miserable when the days are short and dark but perks up when sunnier, warmer weather arrives, it is worth considering this possibility.

Symptoms can be alleviated with the help of medication and light therapy. A winter holiday in a sunnier location will also help if you can manage it, but you can also encourage your child to play outside in the snow on bright days.

SIGNS OF DEPRESSION

As children approach puberty, they invariably suffer mood swings due to the normal hormonal changes that are taking place, so don't automatically assume depression. However, your child may be depressed if he:

- Is lethargic and shows no inclination to play with friends
- Develops an erratic pattern of sleep
- Has bad dreams or nightmares
- Suddenly becomes extremely picky about food
- Begins to perform badly at school
- Displays no enthusiasm for anything.

concerned. Some people believe that a child cannot suffer from real depression, but there is plenty of evidence that children as young as 7 years old are so unhappy that they have contemplated suicide, although suicide itself is rare under the age of 12.

Helping a depressed child

There are several things you can do to help your child. First, you should ensure him that he will always have your love and support. Regularly set aside time especially for him – turn off the television or the radio – and ask him to tell you about his day. It's important for him to know that you are a good listener and are always there for him when he needs to talk. Regular talks will encourage him to tell you when he does have any worries.

Even if you think that his problem is trivial, maybe even laughable, you should always take his distress seriously or your child may never have the confidence to confide in you again. Be aware that an older child may prefer to talk to someone other than you – perhaps a grandparent, uncle, aunt, teacher or even the parent of

a friend. If that is so, try hard not to feel hurt – your child may be trying to protect you from his own unhappiness. The important thing is that he is able to talk to someone.

Outside help

If your child's depression persists, it is time to seek help outside the home. Take him to see his family doctor, who will refer him the to appropriate specialist. Family therapy or counselling is usually the initial type of help offered. The child is seen with all the other members of his immediate family so that the therapist can observe how they interact with each other and learn more about what part the troubled child plays in the family dynamics.

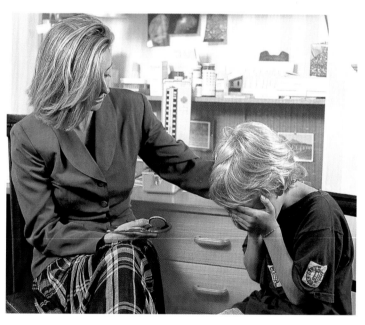

If the root of the problem is seen to be within the child himself, he may be referred to a child psychologist or psychotherapist for counselling on his own. The specialist will try to bring your child's thoughts and emotions to the surface and help him to understand why he is feeling so unhappy.

SEE ALSO

Headaches	**166**
Sleeping problems	**184–185**
Stress and bullying	**186–187**
Eating problems	**190–191**

Seeking help

It is often the child's doctor who diagnoses depression. She can refer him to a counsellor or psychotherapist or suggest family therapy.

Eating problems

Most parents worry about their child's eating habits and diet. Whether it's a baby refusing everything but pasta or an older child with an insatiable appetite for junk food, eating is one issue that frequently causes anxiety.

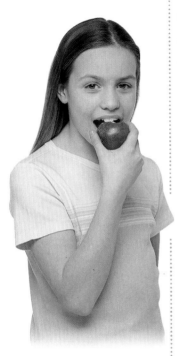

Healthy fast foods
Fresh fruit is an ideal snack food for children. If your child becomes hungry between meals, instead of biscuits or crisps, offer her a choice of fruit from a well-stocked bowl.

From the minute she starts eating solid food, most parents begin to worry about their child's diet. If their baby will only take a certain food and rejects all others, they become anxious that her diet is not varied. However, becoming obsessed about your child's diet may only inhibit her natural curiosity about food.

Iron deficiency anaemia is common in children between six months and two years old. The key to a healthy diet and your child getting enough nutrients is variety and moderation (see p.34). It doesn't make you a less caring parent if you serve commercially prepared food, but you should try to include some home-cooked meals, which will allow your child to experience different textures and tastes.

Selective eating habits

If your child is a faddy eater, you will overcome this problem more quickly by remaining calm and ignoring the fact that for two weeks she has only eaten potatoes. Allow her to have her way, but make a point of sitting down as a family to let her see everyone else eating a healthy variety.

If she has friends who you know eat a varied diet, invite them to play and eat so your child will observe her peers eating normally. Above all, keep a sense of balance – there is no evidence to suggest that young children who have a slightly unconventional diet suffer later on, and it is important that your child adopts a sensible attitude to food and its role.

Junk food

As your child grows older she will be bombarded by junk food. Many schools serve what they know will be eaten and sweets and high-fat foods are still chosen as treats by many families. You cannot prevent your child from trying junk food unless you ban her from birthday parties, visiting friends and socializing in general.

If you know your child has an allergy to certain foods, then tell the parent of the friend she is visiting, but otherwise remain silent. If your daughter asks you

---

A BALANCED DIET

By eating a balanced diet (see p.34), your child will get all the nutrients that she needs to become a healthy adult.

- Proteins build and maintain strong bones. They are found in eggs, milk, cheese, fish, meat, seeds and pulses.
- Carbohydrates, found in cereals, bread, rice, pasta, potatoes, fruit and vegetables, will maintain a balanced metabolism. (These foods also have fibre, which children should not overload on – avoid giving children too many wholemeal products.)
- Minerals and vitamins are needed in small amounts to ensure overall health. They are found naturally in all the above foods, so your child does not need to take supplements.
- Some fat is necessary to insulate against cold and give energy. It can be found in dairy products, nuts, meat, oily fish, cakes and biscuits.

WHAT IS TOO THIN?

If either you or your partner is naturally thin, than you shouldn't be surprised if your child has inherited a slim build. However, if the answer to any of the questions on the right is yes, it may be worth taking her to your doctor, who will be able to keep a check on her weight and height to ensure that all is well.

- Is your child a lot thinner than her peers?
- Has she been wearing the same size clothes for several years?
- Does she always leave food on her plate at mealtimes?
- Is she often tired and listless?
- Does she fall ill a lot?

to buy "treats" because friends will be coming to play, suggest that they make some fruit cakes or biscuits (with your supervision, of course). They will enjoy eating them more than bought items and have fun making them too. As an added bonus, the more you involve your child in cooking, the more likely it is she'll become adventurous with food and have a healthy attitude to eating later on.

The overweight child

If your child is obviously overweight, you should take a look at family life as a whole. Overweight children have a more difficult time at school than their thinner peers, and they find sports difficult, which prepares them for a sedentary, unhealthy adult life. If you are overweight, you may want to improve your own sense of wellbeing, and doing so to help your child may be the incentive you need.

If meal times are quick fixes in front of the television, gradually change the routine. Encourage your child to help plan meals, then together make a list of what you need to buy. When shopping, don't let her persuade you to stray from your shopping list and buy unwholesome items. If sweets and crisps are big in her life, you can gently introduce healthier alternatives. Never place a child on a diet unless under doctor's advice.

Cooking together
Encouraging your child from an early age to help prepare meals is one way to ensure that she will understand and enjoy healthy eating when she becomes an adult.

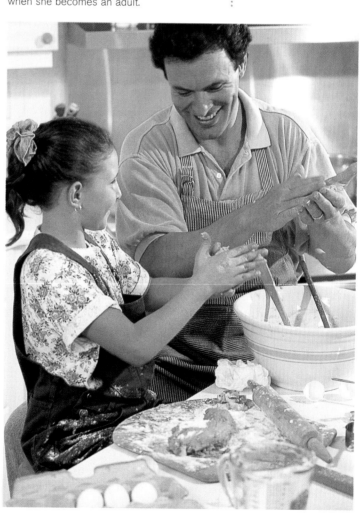

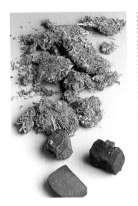

Illegal drugs

Preteen children may try marijuana (above); older children may try Ecstasy, amphetamines, cocaine or heroin. Signs of taking drugs are changes in friends, mood, school performance or sleeping habits – but these could be normal behaviour. Drug paraphernalia, such as cigarette papers or pipes, are clear clues.

Substance abuse

The possibility of your child taking illicit drugs, drinking alcohol, smoking cigarettes or abusing solvents is most parents' nightmare; however, it can happen – and sometimes it must be seriously considered.

Drugs of all kinds have a high profile in modern society, but adolescent children are most likely to experiment with legal, socially acceptable drugs – cigarettes and alcohol. These drugs affect a child's mind and behaviour and pose a serious threat to his health. These are facts that you should explain to your child in an unemotional, matter-of-fact way.

The nicotine in cigarettes is one of the strongest addictive substances known, and cigarette smoking has a myriad of adverse health effects. The best way to deter children from smoking is by setting an example: don't smoke yourself. He is more likely to want to try it if you smoke.

Preventing alcohol abuse

Too much alcohol can also be damaging to health. However, drinking alcohol in a responsible manner is an established part of adult social life and it's unrealistic to preach complete abstinence to your child. Besides, a complete ban will only make it more attractive. In Great Britain, research has shown that just under half of children have had at least one glass of alcohol well before their teens. Intake increases rapidly in their teens. The reason a child usually gives for drinking is that it makes him feel grown up. Curiosity also plays a large part; why does this mysterious liquid make people so happy and lively?

A child tends to be undiscriminating and will try anything he can find in the drinks cupboard. To remove the mystique and instil sensible drinking habits, you can allow him a small amount of wine – perhaps mixed with water – or beer at family meals, but always under your supervision. While there are safe guidelines for adults, there are none for children because their bodies are still developing. Experimental drinking can lead to severe intoxication in which a child experiences breathing difficulties and even coma and death. He will require immediate hospital treatment.

A preteen talk

Before your child starts smoking or taking drugs, calmly tell him why you disapprove of these activities. Ensure it is a two-way conversation by listening to his point of view.

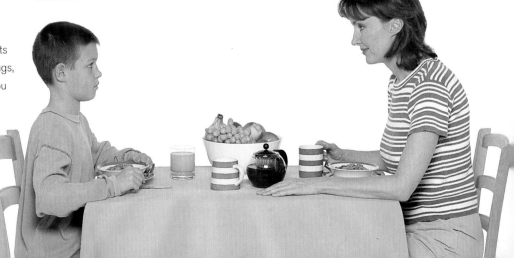

SEE ALSO
Stress and bullying   **186–187**
Depression   **188–189**
Resuscitation (CPR)   **212–215**
Poisoning   **217**

SIGNS OF ABUSE

Some or all of the following symptoms may be evident in a child who has abused drugs or solvents:

- Flushed skin
- Bloodshot eyes
- Dilated pupils
- Vomiting
- A rash around the nose and mouth
- Irritability or a change in personality
- Fatigue
- Uncoordinated movements.

Sniffing solvents

Although solvent abuse mostly happens in the early teens, some younger children do experiment with it, and boys are most at risk. As a parent you may be less informed about such practices than your child, but don't assume that because it is not part of your experience that your child will not be tempted to try it when urged on by his peers. Solvent abuse is usually a group activity. The best way to prevent this kind of experimentation is to have all the facts before you so that you can make him fully aware of the dangers.

Solvents are chemicals that release fumes. Solvent abuse is most commonly referred to as glue sniffing, but there is a wide range of products the abuser can use, many of which are found in the average home (see box, right). When the user inhales the fumes it makes him feel pleasantly light-headed and dreamy; in fact, the experience is similar to being drunk. The less pleasant side effects are dizziness and, possibly, hallucinations; however, these usually wear off quite quickly. The biggest risk is that your child may have an accident while he is under the influence; for example, a number of children have fallen into ponds or rivers and drowned.

Solvent abuse is more dangerous if a child covers his face with a plastic bag in order to maximize the effect – this can quickly lead to unconsciousness. Sometimes, the contents of an aerosol are sprayed directly into the mouth, another dangerous practice, which can make the throat swell, blocking the airways and causing asphyxiation. The use of butane gas can trigger heart failure. Some children have died from choking on their own vomit after indulging in solvent abuse. Most children, however, do not become regular abusers. Those who do persist with the habit run the risk of damaging their brain, liver and kidneys.

Seeking help

If you suspect that your child is indulging in smoking, drinking or drug or solvent abuse try not to panic. Whatever you do, you should not reject him, nor should you pretend that it hasn't happened. Talk to him calmly and rationally, and keep your eyes open for signs that the practice is continuing. For most children this kind of experimentation is a passing phase. However, if you have evidence that your child is a persistent user, you should seek advice from your doctor or contact a family support group.

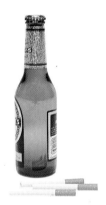

Alcohol and cigarettes
Many children will try alcohol before they reach their teens. Peer pressure is the main reason children begin to smoke cigarettes.

HOUSEHOLD SUBSTANCES

Many of the solvents that children may abuse are readily available in their own home.

Examples include:

- Aerosols
- Metal polish
- Solvent-based adhesives and glues
- Typewriter correction fluid
- Solvent-based marker pens
- Nail varnish remover
- Shoe polish
- Dry cleaning products
- Petrol.

CHAPTER FOUR

Developmental problems and special needs

It is helpful if developmental problems are identified as soon as possible. They may be picked up by parents or during routine health contacts. However, if you believe your child is falling behind his peers in any area – physically or intellectually – do not hesitate to express your concerns to a health visitor or doctor.

Early intervention may reduce the impact of learning difficulties and allow your child to achieve much more than you might have thought possible. For example, it may be a simple matter of organizing special tutoring or fitting a hearing aid that resolves a problem. Sometimes a child who has special needs will do well in a mainstream school – but some children find that they can achieve more in a special school that caters for their particular requirements.

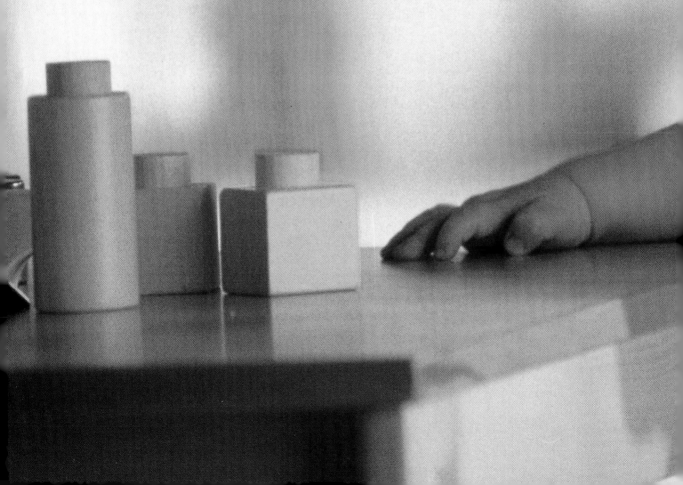

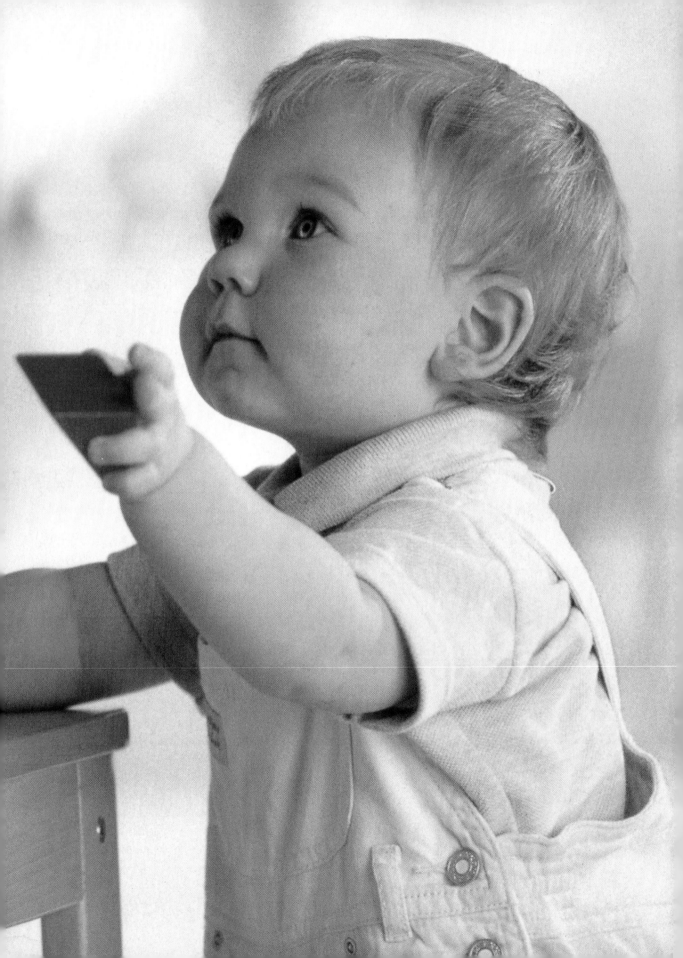

Identifying a child with developmental delay

There is a huge variation in the ages at which children acquire skills, which can make it difficult to know if your child has developmental problems that require attention.

Most parents wait expectantly for each milestone in their child's progress to be reached and often feel disappointed if she does not achieve a new skill or reach a new level of independence at the same age as other children they know. However, just because your baby shows no sign of being able to walk as she approaches her first birthday – although her cousin of the same age is confidently upright – this does not mean that there is a developmental delay. The slow walker has probably found she can move around effectively by crawling. In fact, a normal baby will begin walking at any time between 10 and 18 months. It's much the same with talking. One 18 month old may have a vocabulary with quite a few recognizable words, but your child's vocabulary may be limited to only one or two words.

There are also large differences between how boys and girls develop, something that you should bear in mind when comparing your son with his big sister. If you have only one child, remember that first time parents probably find it more difficult to assess their child than those who have already experienced the way in which children usually progress.

Good coordination

A three year old who can turn the pages of a book is showing signs of developing good coordination.

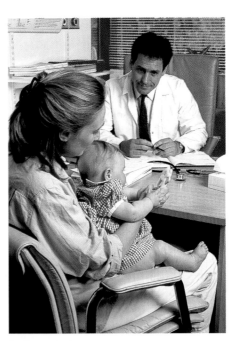

Routine contacts

Your child's progress will be monitored by a health visitor or nurse, with whom you can discuss any concerns that you may have. If a problem is found, she will be referred a doctor.

Slow progresssion

It is only when a child is falling a long way behind all her peers in several areas that parents need to seek advice. Even then, they need to be aware that there are all sorts of factors to be taken into consideration in order to find out why a child is not progressing as quickly as she should do. These include the kind of stimulation she receives at home and from other carers and whether she was born prematurely, has had a serious illness or has undergone some type of trauma such as the breakdown of the family. Even your child's position in the family can have a bearing on the rate of her development.

The eldest child is likely to be far more independent, to be able to dress herself and take herself to the toilet long before the youngest member of the family, who is either too used to having everything done for her to bother to develop self-reliance or whose parents are determined that she should be kept a baby for as long as possible. The youngest child may also be a delayed talker for the simple reason that there is always someone else around to do the talking for her. It does not mean that she doesn't understand everything said, nor that she will never become a sparkling conversationalist.

Always bear in mind that it is only possible for a child to achieve something when the time is right for her, and all the urging in the world will not make her walk confidently or talk fluently before she is ready. Reassure yourself that most children get there in the end.

Getting professional help

There is a small minority of children who do have developmental delay problems, and these children need to be identified as soon as possible. Parents should trust their own instincts when they believe there is something seriously wrong. Too often medical professionals will dismiss parents as just being fussy or overanxious, which means the problem may not be dealt with as early as it should have been.

Early intervention is important in helping to prevent your child from falling further behind. Your doctor should refer her to a specialist for any physical problems that may be hindering her progression such as hearing, speech or visual difficulties (see pp.200–205). She may need special help to proceed with her education if she is delayed mentally.

SEE ALSO
Milestones: newborn
to age 2   **22–23**
Milestones: ages 2–6   **24–25**
Routine health contacts   **30–31**

An alert child
A baby who takes notice of things around him and points is showing an alert, active mind.

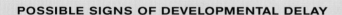

POSSIBLE SIGNS OF DEVELOPMENTAL DELAY

The following may indicate some form of developmental delay:

- Little or no apparent interest or curiosity about the world around her and lack of any significant response to her parents or siblings.

- Poor concentration – nothing seems to keep her attention for more than a few seconds, even the most attractive toy.

- Poor verbal communication – if by the age of 18 months, your child does not have a few recognizable words, even if most of what she says is not yet intelligible.

- Delayed toilet training – by the age of three years, most children are dry and clean during the day, although they may still require nappies at night. If your child still wears nappies 24 hours a day when it's time for her to go to nursery, you should have a word with your doctor, initially to eliminate any physical cause (see pp.156–157).

- Poor manipulative skills – by her first birthday your child should be able to pick up small objects, and by 18 months she is usually able to hold a pencil or thick crayon and make some kind of mark on paper.

- An inability to interact in any way with other children at playgroup or nursery.

Caring for a child with special needs

All children need nurturing by their parents, and although a child with a disability may need additional help, you will feel the same love for him that you would for any child.

Parents whose child has a permanent disability – whether physical or mental – often have to go through a grieving process before they can come to terms with the situation. Everyone has plans for his or her child's future, everyone wishes for healthy children who will perform well at school and become independent, successful adults.

It can, of course, be devastating to discover that your child will not progress at the same rate or be able to achieve the same level of independence as other children. The outlook can suddenly seem very dismal and it is perfectly normal for parents to grieve for the type of child they thought they would have. Only then can they readjust their expectations and set out to provide the kind of life in which their child is able to reach his potential in his own special way.

One of the best ways to overcome your fears of the future is to find out as much as you possibly can about your child's condition. You can start by contacting other parents who have children with the same impairment. This will help you establish the right balance between too high and too low expectations – and it will help alleviate the isolation you may inevitably feel. There is a wide range of voluntary groups that can provide you with this kind of support.

Making adjustments

Above all, it is important to concentrate on your child as a person rather than on his condition and to resist attributing everything that goes wrong in his life to his disability. However severe his needs, you should always remember that he is still an individual in his own right and, as far as possible, you should treat him the same as any other child.

In the early years, it is the parents who are their child's main educators and this doesn't alter because your child has special needs. A special child needs to be talked to and played with just as any other child, and he needs as many toys and books to

Public awareness
Efforts are being made to make more buildings and other facilities accessible to everyone, including those confined to wheelchairs.

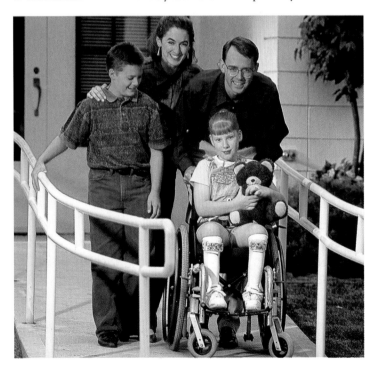

stimulate him and help him to develop new skills. The difference is that they may have to be appropriate for his mental abilities rather than his chronological age. Of course, some specialist help should be available to you, too. One of the most effective is the Portage scheme (so called because it began in Portage, Wisconsin, in the United States), in which a trained home visitor calls on a regular basis to work with parents and children.

As a parent, it will be easy to become overprotective of your child; however, even a child with severe special needs should be allowed to have some involvement in the decisions made about him. This may be a simple matter of offering him some choices about what he eats or what clothes he wears. Allowing him these decisions will help him to feel he has some control over his life.

There is a danger that the child with special needs will be overindulged – a natural reaction from parents who feel their child has been given a raw deal when it comes to life opportunities. But here, too, he needs to be treated, as much as possible, in the same way as his healthy brother or sister. He needs boundaries just as much as they do, and he should expect to be disciplined in an appropriate way if he oversteps the mark.

Outside the home

As a child with special needs grows up, the thing uppermost in a parent's mind is the kind of education he will receive. Will he be able to cope in a mainstream school or will he be happier at a special school that may be better able to serve his needs? The decision will be based on the severity of his learning difficulties, but sometimes parents find that they have to fight for the right education for their child. If you truly believe that professional decisions

are the wrong ones, you have the right to protest. This is not always easy for parents who are naturally quiet or withdrawn people, but often they find inner strength when it comes to fighting for what they believe is best for their child.

If you are ready to battle with teachers, social workers or other professionals, know beforehand what your rights are and always be assertive, not aggressive. However, you must also be prepared to accept decisions you don't like. It may be that you are still in denial about your child's condition and have not yet come to terms with his limitations.

For the child who is physically or mentally different from other children, the outside world is often a harsh one. People can be insensitive and may make unkind comments. Such reactions are usually based on ignorance or fear, but your child should be prepared for them. Before he goes to nursery or to school, try to explain to him that the other children will probably be curious about his wheelchair or the fact that he is slower or moves differently from them. After a bad day when he is feeling hurt and upset, it's important that he feels able to discuss his feelings with you and knows that you will always love and support him.

SEEKING HELP

Contacting a support group can help you cope with your situation. National telephone numbers are listed below. To find a group in your area, look for a number in your local telephone directory.
- Handicapped Adventure Playground Association (HAPA) 0207 731 1435
- National Portage Association 01935 471 641
- National Association of Toy Libraries 0207 387 9592
- Royal Society for Mentally Handicapped Children and Adults (MENCAP) 0207 454 0454
- Council for Disabled Children 0207 843 6061
- Contact a Family 0207 383 3555

Speech and language problems

Difficulties with speech and language development are increasingly common – if your child is referred to a speech therapist, there should be no cause for alarm.

In the ordinary course of events, children will begin to name some objects that they often encounter, as well as coin their own words for other items that they don't know, by the time they are one year old. By two years of age, they will be able to put several words together and chatter to themselves and you, using semi-intelligible language. They may also, at this stage, echo what you say and use pronouns such as "I", "me" and "you".

By the time children turn three years old, they usually may begin joining words, using "with", "from" and "into" to make sentences. Some children are also able to learn and recite simple rhymes by

heart. However, not all children follow this pattern of developing language skills. If your child has not shown any signs of following it, she is only one of a large minority and you should not be overly concerned about her speech.

Changes in the home

There are various theories to try to explain why there has been such a huge increase in speech difficulties in recent years, and the two most common ones are linked to changes in family life. The prominent theory is that young children now spend a considerable amount of time in the company of the television. If the parents are watching it, then they are less likely to be conversing with their child; and if the child is in front of the television, then she is less likely to be talking to her parents.

In addition to the constant sound from the television, there is the bombardment of additional noise from other household appliances, such as washing machines, radios and telephones, which may interfere with listening and speaking skills. So, as a primary measure, it is a good idea to ensure that you set aside some time each day when everything is turned off and you can sit quietly and communicate with your child.

Many twins are late to talk, perhaps because adult attention is always shared between them, and one twin is usually

LISPS, STAMMERING AND STUTTERING

Lisping is characterized by the pronunciation of "s" and "z" sounds as "th". This is usually a temporary stage, often when the first teeth have fallen out and the second teeth have yet to grow. In some cases the child may also affect a lisp because she has a close friend who has one or she realizes it is an attention-grabber. Sometimes it can signify a cleft palate or deafness; if you are worried about the cause, seek the opinion of a speech therapist.

Stammering involves hesitant and interrupted speech. It is more common in boys, as well as in large families where members are competing for attention and a part in the conversation. If the stammer is persistent or interferes with a child's everyday life, seek the advice of a speech and language therapist.

Stuttering is when the same sounds are repeated several times. If it occurs occasionally, it may be the outward sign of your child's brain racing ahead of her ability to form the words. If it happens frequently, seek the advice of a speech and language therapist. Usually, if the child is not teased and the problem is not highlighted, and you listen patiently, she will grow out of it without treatment.

will be given – for example, your child may have to practise blowing on a small ball, which will help her learn how to control air pressure in her mouth. A child who is deaf or partially deaf, must have treatment for that particular problem by a specialist. All other problems can usually be treated directly by a speech therapist.

If your child is saying absolutely nothing at all or speaks only occasionally by the time she is four years old, she may be exhibiting elective mutism – she is able to speak but is choosing not to. This is a rare situation, and it is often attributed to some type of psychological trauma. She will need to see a child psychologist to deal with the emotions that are causing her silence.

Getting help from a therapist

Speech therapy is often successful, and the earlier it is started the better the results will be. If your child stutters, lisps or says nothing at all by the age of two, you should consult your doctor or health visitor about getting a referral to a speech and language therapist. Similarly, if your child's speech is unclear or incomprehensible, you should seek professional help.

Technological help

Some children who do not have the ability to speak can still communicate with others by using computer technology.

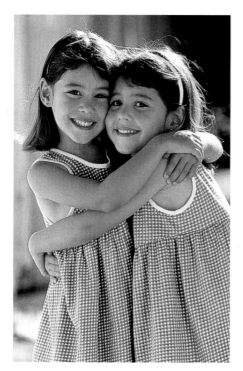

Sharing their own language

Twins often create a special language between themselves, which adults cannot share; so they spend most of the time talking to each other and not to others.

more dominant and takes the lion's share of the attention, as well as speaking for her twin. Sometimes they invent their own language. However, they understand what others say to them and develop normal speech in due course.

Other causes

In some rare cases, damage is done to a part of the child's brain at or before birth, which affects her ability to speak. Speech difficulties can also arise from deafness or partial deafness or from a cleft palate.

Whatever the roots of the problem, it can usually be dealt with and remedied. A cleft palate will require corrective surgery, but it achieves excellent results. After the surgery, speech therapy sessions

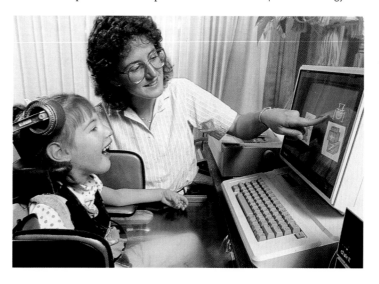

Hearing difficulties

Profound deafness is very rare, but many children suffer from partial hearing loss at some time in their lives and prompt treatment is necessary to avoid speech and developmental problems.

There are two types of deafness. Nerve deafness entails damage to the nerve that carries impulses from the ear to the brain for interpretation. This may be caused by prematurity, rubella during pregnancy (see p.71) or other infectious causes and genetically inherited diseases. The other, more common, type, known as conductive hearing loss, is caused by an infection or a build-up of fluid in the middle ear; it can be effectively treated.

Even when a baby is born profoundly deaf, it may not be noticed before he leaves hospital. When a child is found to have impaired hearing he will need special help and schooling. A child with partial hearing is more difficult to identify, which is why you should always take your child for routine contacts and seek advice from a health visitor if you are concerned about his hearing, understanding or speech. Hearing problems can develop at any stage, but once your child is at school, it is harder to detect a loss of hearing. Children are adept at concealing the problem by relying on friends – copying instructions or asking them to repeat what has been said. If your child has the television volume up loud, seems to guess what you say or becomes withdrawn, ask his teacher to monitor his classroom responses. Make a doctor's appointment if necessary.

Testing a child's hearing

Babies less than six months old are tested in a way that doesn't rely on their cooperation. There are several methods and, in all of them, the response to a special noise is measured with a computer. The results will indicate if the child has a significant hearing loss. If so, further tests may be arranged and, if appropriate, a hearing aid fitted. Babies only a few months old can benefit from them.

For a young child who is able to sit, the distraction test is used. Your child sits on your lap and a trained person sits in front of you. This person will observe your baby's responses to sounds made by a second person behind you. The sounds used may include a mixture of voice sounds, specially designed rattles and artificially produced sounds. If your child fails the test, a repeat test may be arranged after an interval or your child may be referred to a specialist.

An older child can be tested with headphones, through which a painless,

Hearing test

If your child is suspected of having a hearing problem, no matter how young he is, he will have a hearing test. The type of test given will depend on his age.

HEARING AIDS

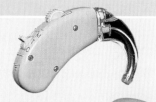

It is unlikely that the hearing aid your child first wears will be so small as to be unseen by others, but a young child is more likely to worry about a hearing aid if gets in the way of play or feels uncomfortable. This is why it is vital, right from the start, to ensure he gets a comfortable fit.

If your child has vision problems as well, you may be able to have a hearing aid that fits on his glasses so that, in effect, there is only one item for him to look after. It is important that his teacher knows how to fit the hearing aid correctly, in case it is removed at school. It is also important that you follow advice given about the care and maintenance of the hearing aid. In a small number of children, it is possible to fit a cochlear implant (an artificial ear).

SEE ALSO

Milestones: newborn to age 2	22–23
The ears and eyes	84–85
Ear problems	86–87

pure tone sound at a chosen pitch is sent into one ear. Young children will be encouraged to indicate whether they can hear by putting a toy into a box. The volume of sound is decreased and a graph is plotted to indicate how much can be heard. The information helps determine the appropriate treatment.

Helping the child

A partially deaf child will need support at school, but he will be able to attend mainstream schools. Speech therapy may be necessary (see pp.200–201) and he may have to wear a hearing aid. If his hearing problem is caused by recurrent ear infections, he will need medical treatment; however, the problem will eventually be resolved and full hearing restored.

Even if a child has a hearing problem, it does not mean that he won't be able to communicate with others. He can be taught sign language and how to read lips. Some people are so adept at reading lips that it's difficult to tell they cannot hear. You can help your child by:

- Buying toys that vibrate when shaken.
- Conversing with him frequently and waiting patiently for him to answer.
- Ensuring he gets the extra support he needs in nursery and school.

- Encouraging others to speak directly to your child; don't answer for him – he needs to learn to communicate for himself.
- Making others aware that deafness does not indicate a lack of intelligence in your child. People sometimes behave in a less enlightened way toward deaf people than they do to people with other disabilities.

Communicating with hands
Sign language is an effective way of communicating and teaching. It can be learned by the deaf person, as well as by his family and friends.

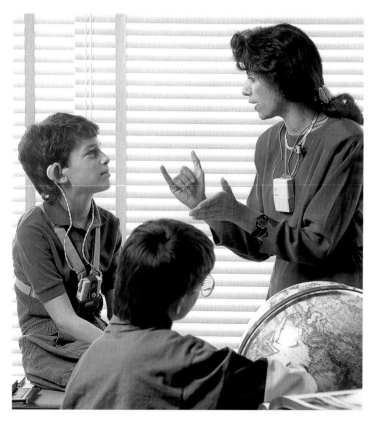

Visual problems

The impairment of sight so common among adults usually begins at some stage during childhood. However, prompt treatment can curtail the problem and ensure that children are free to enjoy an active life.

A new view on life

A child who has not been able to see may suddenly enjoy reading or watching a sporting event once he is fitted with his new glasses.

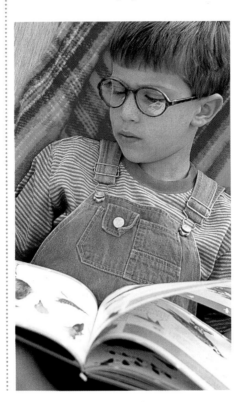

A child's sight can go wrong in a number of ways – whether it be the muscles supporting the eyes, the physical structure of the eye or the ability of the brain to receive nerve impulses from the eye. Routine check ups during both childhood and adulthood are necessary to ensure the eyes function properly.

A squint, or strabismus, is the most common vision problem in babies and young children. It occurs when the muscles attached to an eye are not correctly balanced, so one eye converges or diverges from the other. Some babies are born with a squint, which is inherited, others appear as if they have a squint because of the wide bridge of their nose. Many babies squint while their eye muscles are strengthening.

Squinting should not be ignored once a baby is beyond three months, because it could lead to more serious eye problems. You should seek a prompt consultation with your doctor and referral to an ophthalmologist. Some older children can develop temporary squints, usually caused by overtiredness or anxiety. Treatment for a squint may involve temporarily wearing a corrective eye patch or, in serious cases, surgery.

Cataracts are a much rarer problem for newborn babies – they may be caused by infection during the pregnancy or during birth. The cataract appears as a mistiness over the lens and may be corrected by an operation.

GLASSES VS. CONTACT LENSES

Many children go to great lengths to lose or "forget" to wear their glasses. Try telling your child that if the glasses are worn to correct a problem, there is a possibility that she may grow out of it. It is important to ensure that your child wears the glasses prescribed; otherwise she could put herself at a disadvantage or even in danger because of her weak sight. Sensitivity is called for, plus access to a choice of attractive frames. The glasses should fit comfortably, without pinching the noise or rubbing on the ears.

Contact lenses may be the answer for a child who refuses to wear glasses, especially if she enjoys sports; however, lenses require careful handling and a scrupulous hygiene routine to avoid infection. They are not suitable for young children, but for an older child it is worth discussing the different types available with a specialist.

Other impairments

When the eye itself is not formed properly, this can cause problems focusing. Long-sightedness entails not being able to see clearly objects that are close up. Your child may screw up her eyes to look at books. You may notice her rubbing her eyes a lot, which can cause the eyelids to become inflamed. Your child will need to see an optician, who will prescribe her glasses.

Short-sightedness is a difficulty in focusing on objects a long way off. If your child is affected, you will notice she fails to recognize familiar people and objects from far away; older children will be unable to read bus numbers from a distance and may complain of headaches above the eyes. Young children may try to compensate by looking out of the corner of their eyes to bring objects into focus.

Colour blindness is not uncommon in its mildest form and affects a great many more boys than girls – about 8 percent of boys are affected to some degree. The most usual form is that of being unable, or finding it difficult, to distinguish between the colours red and green. If you notice your child is taking a long time to learn his colours, it may be because he is colour blind. Simple, patient repetition and constant reinforcement when you are on outings and chatting in the home may help him overcome it. Colour blindness is usually not an impediment, apart from excluding a few obvious careers in adulthood.

Blindness

Although very rare, blindness can be caused by diseases either contracted during pregnancy or genetically inherited, or by injury or infection at birth or later in life. Other problems, such as cataracts and severe squints, can deteriorate into blindness if they remain untreated; however, it is unlikely that they would be overlooked by the medical professionals involved at the birth and afterward.

Toxocara canus is another cause of blindness, which affects children in particular because of the way in which it is contracted. *Toxocara canus* is the worm present in dogs that have not been wormed. It is passed on through faeces and so can be picked up by children playing in parks and places where dog owners have been less than responsible. While it is pointless to become obsessional, you should make sure your child is aware from an early age that she must always wash her hands carefully after playing in the park, that she should never lick her hands until she has done so and she should never go near or touch dog faeces.

A child who is blind will require special schooling and support; however, she will be able to function as an independent adult. In fact, there are many inspirational role models to show how much can be achieved by those who are blind.

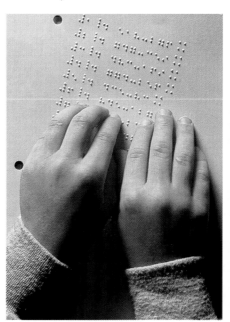

SEE ALSO
Routine contacts 30–31
Infectious diseases 60–61
The ears and eyes 84–85
Eye problems 88–89

Doing homework
Braille, a system of raised dots for each letter in the alphabet and for numbers, allows a blind person to "read". Here, a blind child is reading his mathematics homework.

Learning difficulties

In many cases, a child's learning difficulties are not identified until he begins formal schooling. It's only then that it becomes apparent that his ability to learn is significantly behind that of most children of his age.

Some parents expect their child to start reading and writing as soon as he starts school and panic if he doesn't. They may even be keen to have a learning disability diagnosed when, in fact, none exists. Intellectual ability depends not only on the structure of the brain but also on adequate nutrition, good physical health and an emotionally stable and stimulating environment. This means that children begin school at different levels, and much depends on the kind of preschool experience they have had.

A child who has been in a nursery school for a year is likely to appear more forward than a child who has not had that advantage. The child whose parents have instilled in him an enthusiasm for

learning and have provided him with a lot of books, as well as writing and drawing materials, is likely to make good progress, at least at the initial stage. Some children start school already able or ready to read, yet others may take several years to reach the same level; however, in time, they will become equally fluent.

The age at which a child starts school does not necessarily have any influence on when he becomes a fluent reader. Indeed, some people believe that an early start can have a negative effect on the child and lead to reading failure. In Europe, children begin formal learning as young as four and a half and as late as seven years old. It has been found that there is no absolute link between the level

Learning by computer

Many schools now provide computers for children to learn on. Those with learning difficulties can often do well with this teaching tool.

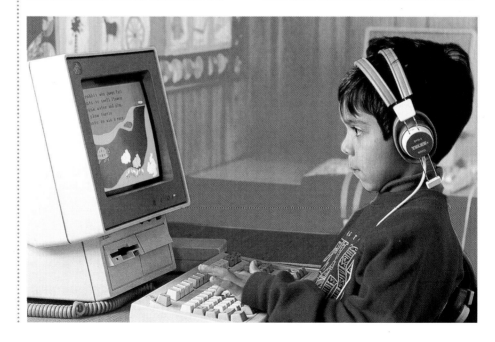

of literacy at the age of nine and the time the child started schooling. Some experts believe that a mental age of six to six and a half is the optimal age for the teaching of reading to begin.

A child may be some months into his first year at school before a learning disability is identified. Once a teacher is familiar with him and his capabilities, she will be able to judge whether he is progressing at the same rate as his peers or is falling far behind in one or more areas of the curriculum.

The child's education

A learning difficulty can be defined as mild, moderate or severe. Mild and moderate forms are most common, and children with these forms are able to remain in mainstream education, with the benefit of some extra help until the problem is overcome. When a child has a severe learning difficulty, it is concluded that he is unable to benefit from the usual kind of educational facilities for children of his age and he is given a place at a special school that can be more sensitive to his individual needs.

Research has shown that one in five children will have some kind of special educational need at some point in their school lives. However, it's important to bear in mind that complete failure to learn is unusual. Both parents and teachers should be aware that a learning problem can usually be reversed and, if appropriate action is taken at the right time, the problem may be overcome. The expectations of both parents and teachers can affect a child's progress, so they need to be careful not to place too much emphasis on one specific learning difficulty, which can risk damaging his confidence so much that he begins to fail in other areas as well.

Dyslexia

One type of specific learning disability is dyslexia, in which a child cannot process symbolic information such as the letters in words. It occurs more frequently in boys than in girls. A dyslexic child is usually of at least average intelligence and is likely to be just as able as his peers in areas other than literacy. He tends to have good verbal skills and is often talented in art or music. However, he will read slowly and with a lack of comprehension, and he will usually make peculiar errors and omissions in reading and spelling.

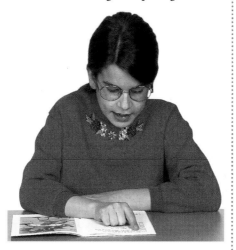

It is important for the diagnosis to be made as soon as possible. If the problem isn't identified until adolescence, the child will almost inevitably have fallen behind in all academic areas. If your child's school does not seem to be taking his problems seriously, you should insist that he is seen by an educational psychologist.

There isn't a cure for the condition, but a dyslexic child can be taught techniques for coping. New technology and the increased use of computers have done much to improve the outlook for him. Although some difficulty with reading and spelling is likely to persist throughout life, many dyslexic people go on to lead successful lives.

SEE ALSO

Milestones: ages 2–6 **24–25**

Shyness and insecurity **174–175**

Identifying a child with developmental delay **196–197**

Reading the print
Some children with dyslexia have trouble seeing black print on white paper, especially under fluorescent lights. Special tinted glasses can help the child read.

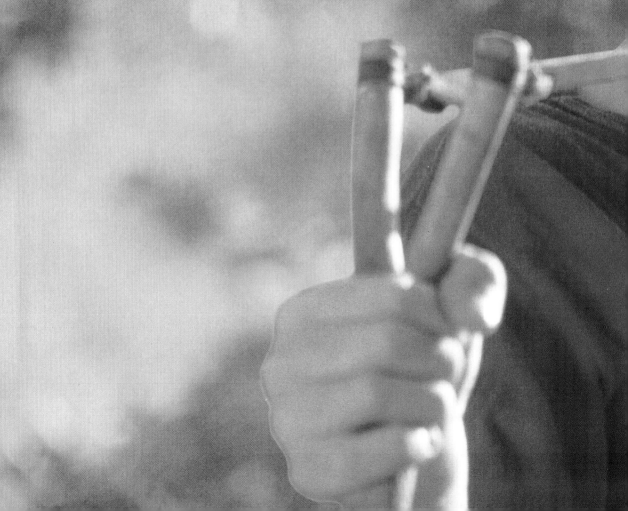

CHAPTER FIVE

Coping with emergencies

Accidents will happen – particularly to young children whose natural exuberance and curiosity often lead them into danger. All parents, even those with "well-behaved" children, can find themselves suddenly coping with a life-threatening situation.

It is important that you have a basic knowledge of first aid. It will boost your self-confidence and, more importantly, help you remain calm and in control should such an emergency arise. The best way to learn first aid is to take a course offered by a professional organization such as the Red Cross. You can find telephone numbers for local chapters of such organizations in your telephone directory.

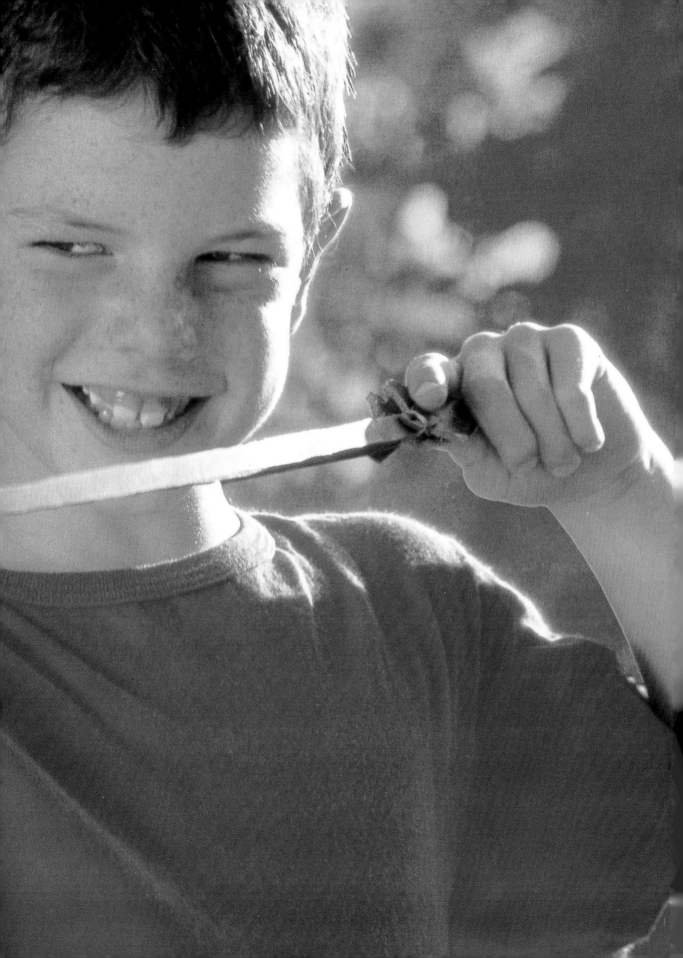

Choking

An object blocking the trachea, or windpipe, causes choking. A child under three years is likely to choke on a swallowed object; in an older child, choking is usually caused by food going down the windpipe.

The symptoms of a baby choking are difficulty in breathing; making odd noises or no sound; and a red face and neck. In a child, the symptoms are difficulty in speaking and breathing; the child's hands rising to her throat; her face turning blue; and the veins in her neck possibly standing out.

REMOVING THE OBJECT

Use your forefinger in a hook shape to remove an object, but never try to remove it unless it is toward the front of the mouth – otherwise you risk pushing it further down the throat.

When helping a child who is choking, after each step:

● Check for an obstruction in the mouth.
● If you cannot remove the obstruction, go to the next step.
● If you remove the obstruction, put a breathing child in the recovery position (see p.213 or p.215).
● If the object is removed but the child is not breathing, give her five artificial breaths (see steps 1–3, p.212 or p.214).

Never leave a baby alone with a bottle or feeding cup or leave a toddler alone with snacks. Never give nuts to a child under five, and don't let a child run about with food, including sweets, in her mouth.

Babies under 1 year old

1 Sitting upright, support the baby over your left forearm (if you are right-handed, or right forearm if you are left-handed). Keep her face down over your knees, with your left hand supporting her chin; her head will be slightly lower than her body. With your free hand, firmly slap between her shoulder blades. Repeat this action five times, checking to see if the object has been dislodged. If not, go on to the next step.

2 Turn the baby face up, supporting her on your knees and using your right hand to support her head. Measure a finger's width below the nipple, then use two fingers to press down firmly to a depth of about 2.5 cm (1 in) five times. Check for a dislodged object. If it still hasn't been freed, repeat steps 1 and 2 three times. If the windpipe is still blocked, call 999 and continue the steps. If your baby loses consciousness, start CPR (see pp.212–213).

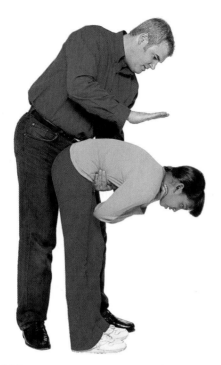

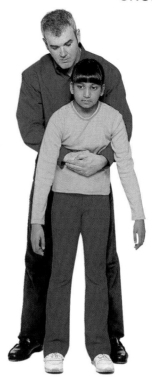

Conscious child

1 Standing behind the child, get her to bend over from the waist (gravity will help dislodge the object), and support her weight with your left hand under her abdomen. Give her five sharp back slaps. If the object hasn't been dislodged, straighten the child and go on to the next step.

2 With a clenched fist, thumb against her abdomen, move your hands midway between the end of her sternum (breastbone) and her navel. Give five sharp thrusts inward. If choking continues, call 999; then repeat the steps. If she loses consciousness, use the method described below.

Unconscious child

1 With the child lying on the floor, roll her on her side toward you and support her head. Give five sharp back slaps. Roll the child on her back and check for a dislodged object. If the object hasn't been dislodged, go on to the next step.

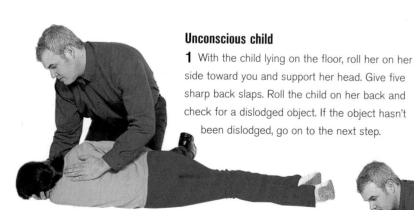

Note: If the child is large, kneel astride her for better positioning of your hands.

2 Place the heel of your hand halfway between her sternum and navel. Place your other hand on top of it; push inward and upward five times. Repeat if the object isn't freed. Feel for a pulse (see step 4, p.214) at intervals; if needed, start CPR (see pp.214–215).

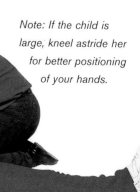

Resuscitation (CPR)

Accidents occur frequently in childhood and occasionally one can be so serious that a child loses consciousness and stops breathing. Knowing how to give cardiopulmonary resuscitation (CPR) in advance could save a child's life.

When a child stops breathing he will become unconscious because no oxygen is able to reach the brain. This lack of oxygen also causes the heart to beat more slowly, and if action isn't taken, the heart will stop altogether. The purpose of resuscitation is to keep the brain alive. The steps involved will provide oxygen to the child's brain and keep his blood circulating until emergency help arrives.

It is a good idea to practise resuscitation before an emergency occurs. The best way to do this is to take a first aid course, where you can learn how to resuscitate with the use of dummies.

The action you should take will differ, depending on whether you are helping a baby under 12 months old (see below) or an older child (see pp.214–215). If a child loses consciousness, send someone to call 999 while you begin CPR. If you are alone, follow the steps for one minute, then call 999 before continuing. Only breathe into a baby or child until his chest rises, then let it fall. If the baby or child starts breathing on his own, put him in the recovery position, which will prevent him from choking or vomiting.

Resuscitating a baby under 12 months old

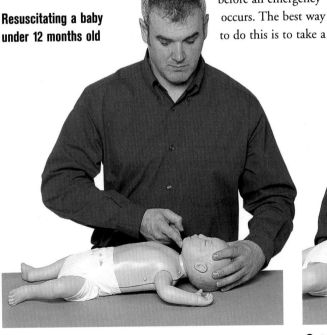

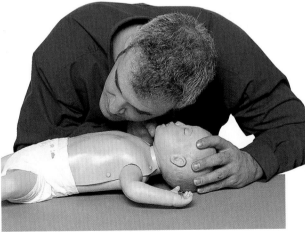

1 Shake him gently and call his name to try to get a response. Lie him on a flat surface. Lift his chin with one finger and tilt his head back slightly to open the airway. Gently supporting the sides of his head, quickly check in his mouth for any obvious obstruction (see p.210).

2 Still supporting his head and keeping his chin raised, lower your cheek toward his nostrils. For 10 seconds, check for breathing by listening for his breath and feeling for it on your cheek. Look along his chest to see if it is rising and falling. If he is breathing, put him in the recovery position.

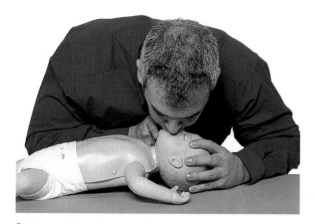

3 If he isn't breathing, cover his mouth and nose with your mouth; breathe into him until his chest rises, then let it fall. Repeat five times; after each breath, observe his chest to see if it rises on its own. If so, put him in the recovery position.

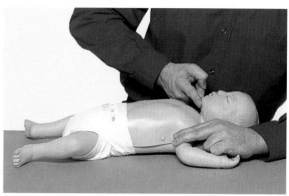

4 After five breaths, feel for his pulse on the inside of the upper arm or in the groin for five seconds; use two fingers flat against the skin. If the pulse is okay but the baby isn't breathing, return to step 3. If there is no pulse, go to step 5.

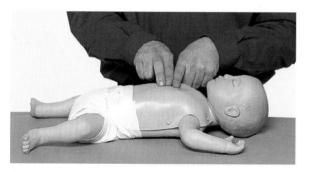

5 To locate where to give chest compressions, measure on the sternum one finger's width below the nipple line. Place two fingertips alongside this finger; remove the first finger. Support the baby's head tilted back with his airway open.

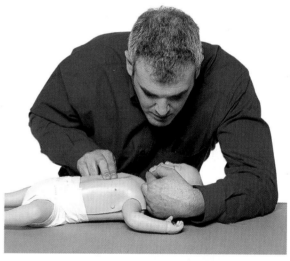

6 Press down five times to 2 cm (¾ in) deep. Repeat the procedure, giving five compressions and one breath every three seconds until help arrives or the heartbeat returns and the baby is breathing – place him in the recovery position.

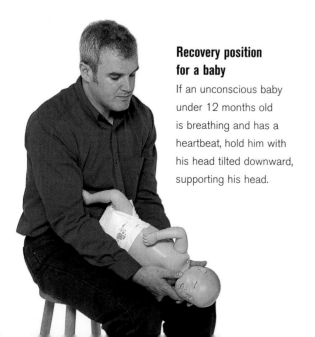

Recovery position for a baby

If an unconscious baby under 12 months old is breathing and has a heartbeat, hold him with his head tilted downward, supporting his head.

ABC CHECK

The letters ABC can help you to remember the steps:
- A is for Airway – keep the airway open by making sure the head is tilted back.
- B is for Breathing – look for the chest rising.
- C is for Circulation – feel for a pulse.

If the child begins breathing at any time, put him into the recovery position.

Resuscitation for older children

The procedures for resuscitating a child over 12 months old follow the basic principles of resuscitating a baby (see p.212), but the steps are adapted for a larger body. Before starting resuscitation, check if the child is unconscious by shaking him gently and asking in a loud voice if he all right. If he responds with a groan, you will know that he is breathing. If there is no response, begin the CPR routine immediately.

Resuscitating a child over 1 year old

1 Lie the child on his back on a firm surface. Put one hand on his forehead, place two fingers of the other hand under his chin and gently tilt back his head to open his airway. Quickly check for any obvious obstruction in his mouth (see p.210).

2 While supporting his head to keep the airway open, check for breathing by listening for it and feeling for it on your cheek. At the same time, look along the line of his chest to see if it is rising. If he isn't breathing, keeping his head tilted back, go on to the next step.

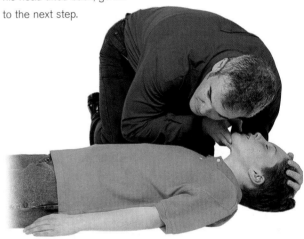

3 Pinch his nostrils to keep them closed. Cover his mouth with your mouth and breathe into him until his chest rises, then let it fall; repeat five times. Take your mouth away after each breath and observe his chest to see if he has begun to breathe again. If he has, put him in the recovery position. If not, go on to the next step.

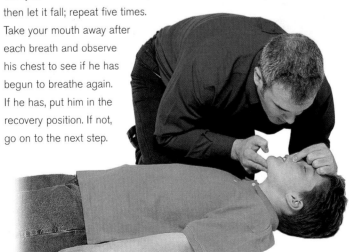

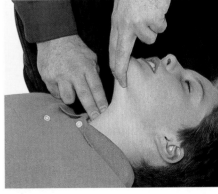

4 Feel for his pulse by pressing two fingers gently on one side of his neck at the carotid pulse. Hold them in place for 10 seconds. If you can't find a pulse, go on to the next step. If you can, go back to step 3.

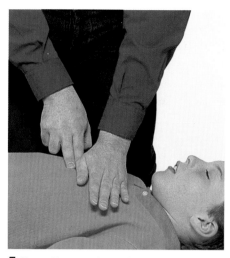

5 To position your hands for compressions, measure two fingers' width from the bottom of his breastbone and place the heel of the other hand by them; for a child over seven years old, link your hands together (see right).

6 Keeping your arm(s) straight, firmly press down 2.5 cm (1 in) deep, five times; give a breath. Repeat the steps for a minute; call 999. Start over again: for a child between one and seven years, give five compressions and one breath every three seconds; for a child over seven, every six seconds. Check the pulse every minute. Continue until help arrives or the heartbeat and breathing start and you can put the child in the recovery position.

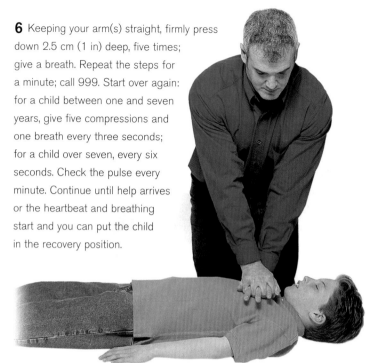

Putting a child into the recovery position

1 Open the airway (see step 1, opposite). Gently lift the arm furthest away from you and bring it across his chest. Put his hand, palm open, against his cheek. Bend the knee furthest away from you, and let his foot rest flat on the ground.

2 Make sure his hand is still pressed against his cheek while you roll him over gently on to his side. Let him rest against your knees to prevent him from flopping on to the ground.

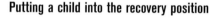

3 Gently rest him on the ground, with the top knee bent. Check that his airway is open and his chin is resting on his palm.

Burns

It is vital to act fast when a child has been burned. Immerse the affected area in cool water for 10 minutes. The water doesn't have to be icy, just cool enough to reduce the temperature of the skin and minimize injury. If the child has clothing on the affected area that can be removed easily without causing pain, then do so; but if there is a risk of pulling at damaged skin, do not touch it. Remove any belts and jewellery in case the area swells up.

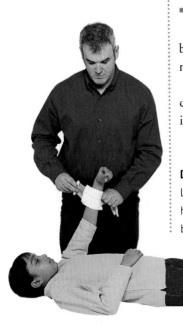

Applying dressing to a burn
Lie the child down and raise the wound. Apply a dressing – in this case, cling film.

To keep a small burn clean, loosely cover it with cling film or a nonfluffy dressing. A burn may blister (see p.105); do not burst it because it may become infected. Consult a doctor if the burn is more than 30 mm (1¼ in) in diameter.

A large burn may cause shock and needs immediate medical attention. Loosely cover it with cling film; apply cling film lengthwise to allow room for swelling. Lightly bandage it in place if needed, but leave room for air to circulate to aid healing. Take the child to a hospital.

SHOCK

The signs of a child going into shock are a pale face, clammy, cold skin and shallow breathing. Lay her down, raise her legs 30 cm (12 in), cover her with a blanket and call 999.

Bleeding

To treat a nosebleed, sit the child with her head between her legs. To help the blood clot, if she can breathe through her mouth, pinch the nostrils for 10 minutes.

For a minor wound apply a clean dressing to the area and place pressure on it to stop the bleeding. If there is glass or

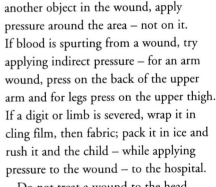

Dressing a cut
Lie the child down and raise the wound above her body. Apply a dressing, using pressure, but not so tight that circulation stops.

another object in the wound, apply pressure around the area – not on it. If blood is spurting from a wound, try applying indirect pressure – for an arm wound, press on the back of the upper arm and for legs press on the upper thigh. If a digit or limb is severed, wrap it in cling film, then fabric; pack it in ice and rush it and the child – while applying pressure to the wound – to the hospital.

Do not treat a wound to the head with pressure, but cover it with a clean dressing and take the child to a hospital. Bleeding from the ears or nose when a head injury is suspected is an emergency. All serious bleeding requires immediate professional help – call 999.

Electric shock

If your child is still touching the source of the electricity, turn off the supply at the mains or use a wooden broom or chair to push her away from the electrical circuit. It is safest to put on rubber boots or stand on a large pile of newspapers or a plastic bin lid to ensure you do not become part of the circuit. As a last resort, without touching the child, grasp any of her loose, dry clothing to pull her away.

You may need to treat your child for burns (see opposite) or resuscitate her (see pp.212–215). If she doesn't need resuscitation but is unconscious, put her in the recovery position (see p.213 or p.215) and call 999 for help.

Poisoning

Young children often mistake unknown substances for familiar items, and their natural curiosity means they will put almost anything into their mouth. Diligence is needed in keeping poisonous items out of their reach (see pp.44–47). An unconscious child may need resuscitating (see pp.212–215).

POISONING

Poison	Symptoms	Treatment
Drugs and alcohol	A child who has swallowed pills or drunk alcohol may be unconscious or may be vomiting, confused and dizzy or have abdominal pain. If stimulants were taken she may be frenzied and sweating; narcotics will make her sluggish.	Do not wait to see if the effects will wear off. If she is able to tell you the cause, or you can quickly locate the bottle, take it with you to the hospital. If you cannot discover the cause but she is vomiting, take a sample of the vomit with you.
Household products	Nail polish remover, corrosive cleaning fluids and bleach have all been known to be drunk by children. You may notice swollen lips, burns around her mouth, bloodstained vomit and difficulty in breathing.	Wipe away any fluid around the mouth and remove any clothing if the fluid has spilled on it. Give her three to four cups of milk to drink before going to the hospital – do not try to make her vomit.
Plants, berries and fungi	Many different berries, leaves and fungi can be deadly. Stomach cramps and vomiting may occur.	Keep the child bent forward to avoid choking if vomiting is severe. Take her to the hospital, along with the plant, berry or mushroom she swallowed. If it is not available, take along any clothes that have been stained by berries or another part of a plant, or take a sample of the vomit.

Broken bones

Most children are extremely active, so it's not surprising that they often suffer from broken bones. If they need to be moved out of the way of danger, you can support the injured limb, or limbs, until help arrives.

Applying traction

If help will be delayed, reduce bleeding and pain with traction: gently but steadily pull on the foot in line with the bone if the child can bear it.

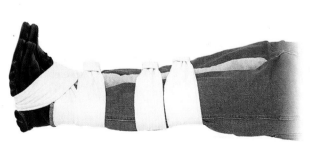

If you know your child has had a fall or accident and notice that she is reluctant to use that part of her body, assume that she may have a broken bone. You may see swelling and redness around the area.

All broken bones require hospital treatment as soon as possible. Take care that moving the child causes no further injury. If injury to the back or neck is suspected, it is best not to move the child unless he will be in danger or needs CPR. If he is in the middle of a road, stop the traffic rather than moving the child. If only a broken arm is suspected, apply a sling or hold the arm in position and take him to a hospital. It is better not to treat a suspected leg fracture but to wait for an ambulance if you can.

Leg splints and arm slings

With leg injuries, if you must move him, grasp him on his uninjured side when you pick him up – try to get someone to help you support him. If the skin is broken and bleeding, raise the limb, if possible, and apply pressure to stop the bleeding (see p.217) but don't press on the bone. When splinting the legs, use towels for padding and any fabric if you don't have bandages.

It is important to support a broken arm. You can improvise a sling with any fabric if you do not have a bandage, or pin a coat or jacket sleeve to hold and support the injured arm.

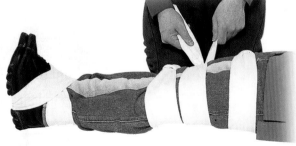

Lower leg splint

If the lower leg is injured, after applying traction, slip two bandages under the knee and another two under the ankle. Place padding between the legs; move the sound leg near the injured one. Tie a figure of eight around his feet; tie the bandages at the knees, then above and below the fracture.

Upper leg splint

After applying traction, ease two bandages under his knees; slide them above and below the injury; ease a bandage under his knees and one under his ankles. Put padding between his legs. Tie a bandage in a figure of eight at the feet; tie the bandage at the knees, then those above and below the injury.

Arm slings

1 Gently ease a triangular bandage or other material under the arm, with the point past the elbow. Bring the side up, with its end around the child's neck. The base of the triangle should run down the front of the child.

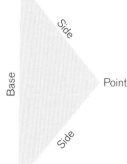

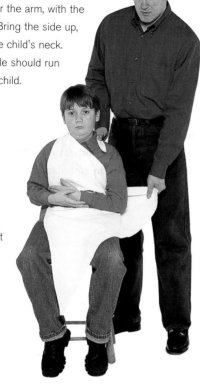

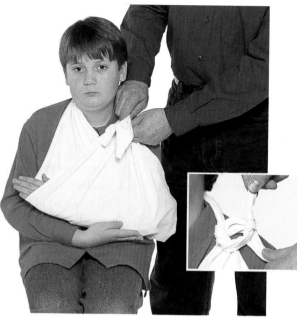

2 Bring the end of the second side up, and tie a reef knot by his collar bone. To tie a reef knot, bring the left end over and under the right one, then the right end over and under the left one. The hand of the injured arm should be raised. The child can support the arm with his free hand.

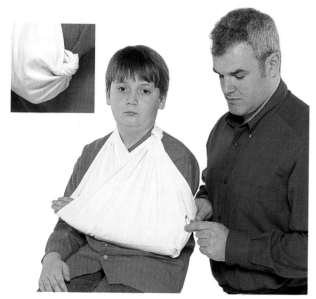

3 Carefully secure the elbow point of the bandage with a safety pin. Tuck in any extra fabric so that it doesn't catch on anything. If a safety pin isn't available, you can twist the end of the fabric and tuck it inside the sling.

HEAD INJURIES

- If you suspect a significant head injury from a blow to the head or fall from a height, call 999 or take the child to the hospital.
- While waiting for help to arrive, if the child is conscious and breathing okay, support his head by holding it aligned with his spine.
- If the child loses consciousness put him in the recovery position (see p.213 or p.215). If his breathing is obstructed, open his airways (see p.212 or p.214); or if there is no breathing or pulse, begin CPR (see pp.212–215).

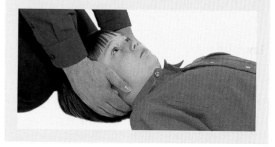

Index

Acknowledgments

Illustrations
All illustrations by Mike Saunders, with the exception of those by Ruth Lindsay (Linden Artists Ltd) on pp.62, 74–75, 83, 132–134, 138, 140, 154, 164–165 and Sally Launder on pp.28–29.

Picture credits
All photographs by John Freeman, with the exception of those listed below.

l=left; *r*=right; *t*=top; *b*=bottom; *c*=centre.
p.2*l* Lori Adamski Peek/Tony Stone Images, 2*r* Bob Thomas/Tony Stone Images; 3*l* Bruce Ayres/Tony Stone Images, 3*r* Adrian Weinbrecht; 6*l* Camille Tokerud/Tony Stone Images, 6*r* Jurgen Magg/Images Colour Library; 6/7 Graem Harris/Tony Stone Images; 7*l* The Stock Market, 7*r* AGE Fotostock/Images Colour Library; 8/9 Camille Tokerud/Tony Stone Images; 10 Bubbles/J Fisher; 12 Anthony Dawton/Bubbles; 13–14 Corbis/Jennie Woodcock, Reflections Photo Library; 15 Laura Wickenden; 16–18 Adrian Weinbrecht; 20 Steven Peters/Tony Stone Images; 21 The Wellcome Trust Medical Photographic Library; 23*r* Laura Wickenden; 26 David De Lossy/The Image Bank; 27*t* George Shelly/Stock Market, 27*b* Paul Barton/Stock Market; 30 Corbis/Jennie Woodcock, Reflections Photol Library; 32 The Stock Market; 35 Laura Wickenden; 36 Adrian Weinbrecht; 39 Laura Wickenden; 40*b* Clarks International; 44 Bubbles/Frans Rombout; 45 Bubbles/Loisjoy Thurston; 47 Alan Danaher/Image Bank; 49*t* The Stock Market, 49*b* Britax Excelsior Ltd; 50*c* Andrew Sydenham; 51 Laura Wickenden; 52*b* Ronnie Kaufman/Stock Market; 53 Andrew Sydenham; 56 Bubbles/Jennie Woodcock; 59 Jurgen Magg/Images Colour Library; 60*t* Bubbles/Jennie Woodcock, 60*b* Corbis/Jennie Woodcock, Reflections Photo Library; 63 Ross Whitaker/Image Bank; 64 The Wellcome Trust Medical Photographic Library; 65 The Stock Market; 66 A B Dowsett/Science Photo Library; 67*r* The Wellcome Trust Medical Photographic Library; 68 Lowell Georgia/Science Photo Library; 69 The Wellcome Trust Medical Photographic Library; 70 Bubbles/Angela Hampton; 71*t* The Wellcome Trust Medical Photographic Library, 71*b* Dr P Marazzi/Science Photo Library; 73 Robert Holland/Image Bank; 75 Jose L Pelaez Inc/Stock Market; 77*t* Mark Clarke/Science Photo Library, 77*b* Asthma Campaign; 78 CNRI/Science Photo Library; 79 Corbis/Bruce Burkhardt; 80 Ken Lax/Science Photo Library; 82 Axair Ltd; 86 Romilly Lockyer/Image Bank; 88 Bubbles/Rohith Jayawardine; 89*t* Dr P Marazzi/Science Photo Library, 89*b* Science Photo Library; 92–97 Bubbles/Jennie Woodcock; 98 Bubbles/Loisjoy Thurston; 102 Dr P Marazzi/Science Photo Library; 103–104 The Wellcome Trust Medical Photographic Library; 106 Dr P Marazzi/Science Photo Library; 107 David Parker/Science Photo Library; 109*l* Milton Reisch/Corbis, 109*b* The Wellcome Trust Medical Photographic Library; 110 Dr P Marazzi/Science Photo Library; 112 R B Studio/Stock Market; 113*t* Science Photo Library; 117 The Wellcome Trust Medical Photographic Library; 122 Paul Barton/Stock Market; 124–125 Professor T Southwood/University of Birmingham; 126 Lawrence Migdale/Tony Stone Images; 127 The Wellcome Trust Medical Photographic Library; 131 Princess Margaret Rose Orthopaedic Hospital/Science Photo Library; 135 ZEFA-Stockmarket; 136 BSIP Laurent/Gille/Science Photo Library; 138 Mark Clarke/Science Photo Library; 139 The Image Bank; 141 Prof K Seddon and Dr T Evans, Queen's University Belfast/Science Photo Library; 142*t* Science Photo Library, 142*b* Gary Parker/Science Photo Library; 144 Dr Ben Oostra/The Wellcome Trust Medical Photographic Library; 145 Richard Gross/Stock Market; 146 Bubbles/Geoff du Feu; 149 Prof Marcel Bessis/Science Photo Library; 151 Optident Ltd; 152 The Stock Market; 153 The Wellcome Trust Medical Photographic Library; 157 David De Lossy/Image Bank; 158 Bubbles/Loisjoy Thurston; 162 CNRI/Science Photo Library; 165 Bubbles/Ian West; 167 Bubbles/Loisjoy Thurston; 168 Dag Sundberg/Image Bank; 169 SCOPE; 171*t* David Pollack/Stock Market, 171*b* Stephen Derr/Image Bank; 172–173 Graeme Harris/Tony Stone Images; 175*t* Bubbles/Frans Rombout, 175*b* Bubbles/Pauline Cutler; 176 Laura Wickenden; 177 Bubbles/Jacqui Farrow; 178 David Oliver/Tony Stone Images; 180 Britt Erlanson/Image Bank; 181 Corbis/Jennie Woodcock, Reflections Photo Library; 182 The Stock Market; 184 Corbis/Jennie Woodcock, Reflections Photo Library; 185*t* Corbis/Paul A Souders; 187 Corbis/Jennie Woodcock, Reflections Photo Library; 188 Bubbles/Jennie Woodcock; 189 Mark Clarke/Science Photo Library; 191 Yellow Dog Productions/Image Bank; 192*t* James King-Holmes/Science Photo Library; 194–195 The Stock Market; 196*r* Jon Gray/Tony Stone Images; 197 Laura Wickenden; 198 Barros and Barros/Image Bank; 201*t* The Stock Market, 201*b* Russell D Curtis/Science Photo Library; 202 CC Studio/Science Photo Library; 203*t* and 203*c* Jane Shemilt/Science Photo Library, 203*b* ZEFA-Stockmarket; 204 The Stock Market; 205 Will and Deni McIntyre/Science Photo Library; 206 Bobbi Lane/Tony Stone Images; 207 Alex Bartel/Science Photo Library; 208 AGE Fotostock/Images Colour Library; 217*b* Corbis/Eric and David Hosking.
Front cover: *t* ZEFA-Stockmarket, *bl* Corbis/Bruce Burkhardt, *bc* The Stock Market, *br* Joe Bator/Stock Market.
Back cover: *t* Laura Wickenden, *bl* Julian Calder/Tony Stone Images, *bc* The Stock Market, *br* CNRI/Science Photo Library.

The publishers are grateful to the following for their assistance in compiling this book: John & Arthur Beare; Children's Liver Disease Foundation; Cystic Fibrosis Trust; Steve Differ; Frances de Rees; Down's Syndrome Association; The Foundation for the Study of Infant Deaths; The National Society for Phenylketonuria (United Kingdom) Limited; Paediatric AIDS Resource Centre; St John Ambulance.